The Herd

Johan Anderberg is a Swedish journalist and writer who has been a regular contributor to a number of Swedish and international media outlets, including *Fokus*, *Sydsvenskan*, and *The Wall Street Journal*. This is his third book.

Alice E. Olsson is a literary translator, writer, and editor working across Swedish and English. She has served as the cultural affairs adviser at the Swedish embassy in London, and during the pandemic has divided her time between Sweden, the UK, and the US.

The Herd

how Sweden chose its own path
through the worst pandemic in 100 years

Johan Anderberg

Translated from the Swedish by Alice E. Olsson

SCRIBE

Melbourne • London

Scribe Publications
2 John St, Clerkenwell, London, WC1N 2ES, United Kingdom
18-20 Edward St, Brunswick, Victoria 3056, Australia
3754 Pleasant Ave, Suite 100, Minneapolis, Minnesota 55409, USA

First published in Sweden by Albert Bonniers Förlag as *Flocken* in 2021

Published by Scribe in 2022

Text copyright © Johan Anderberg 2021
Translation copyright © Alice E. Olsson 2022

Typeset in Adobe Caslon Pro by the publishers

Printed and bound in the UK by CPI Group (UK) Ltd, Croydon CR0 4YY

Scribe is committed to the sustainable use of natural resources and the use of
paper products made responsibly from those resources.

978 1 913348 90 8 (UK edition)
978 1 950354 89 4 (US edition)
978 1 922310 93 4 (Australian edition)
978 1 922586 31 5 (ebook)

Catalogue records for this book are available from the National Library of
Australia and the British Library.

scribepublications.co.uk
scribepublications.com
scribepublications.com.au

To Nora and Elin

Contents

Prologue

On Friday 6 March 2020, three doctors in their sixties arrived at an inconspicuous building on the border between Solna and Stockholm.

It was already late in the afternoon. All day, they had been trying to make the meeting happen. It had been pushed back again and again. But now it was going ahead.

The first doctor was Jan Albert. He was the leader. Albert was a professor in infectious-disease control at the Karolinska Institute. He was the one who had set up the meeting.

The second was Johan von Schreeb. He was the celebrity. Von Schreeb was a storm chaser who would get on a plane as soon as disaster struck anywhere in the world. Way back in 1993, he had founded the Swedish section of Doctors Without Borders; in 2014, he had been named 'Swede of the Year' by the news and current affairs magazine *Fokus*.

The third was Denis Coulombier. He was the Frenchman. Up until the year before, Coulombier had been head of the preparedness and response unit at the ECDC — the European Centre for Disease Prevention and Control, headquartered in Sweden.

Now he was formally retired, but remained an authority.

As they waited inside the offices of the Swedish Public Health Agency, the sky was darkening outside.

Finally, Anders Tegnell, Sweden's state epidemiologist, came to meet them. They sat down in the agency's empty dining hall and began to converse.

Denis Coulombier already knew Tegnell. In his position at the ECDC, he'd met with all the European heads of infectious-disease control on several occasions.

This time, he thought, the Swede looked tired.

Jan Albert was the first to speak: 'There is an opportunity to act now.'

Six days earlier, the February school break had ended in Stockholm.

Many of those who had returned from Italy and Austria had brought back an infection. They were carrying SARS-CoV-2 — a virus originating in China that gave rise to a mysterious pneumonia-like illness.

Jan Albert had helped Region Stockholm forecast the spread of the virus, and what he saw worried him. He told Tegnell about two studies he'd read that seemed to indicate that children could spread the disease even if they weren't exhibiting symptoms. In Spain and Italy, he continued, the rate at which the infection spread was already exponential. Soon it would be here, too.

Johan von Schreeb recounted a few conversations he'd had with colleagues in Italy. Of the patients ending up in hospital, more than one in five needed intensive care.

Then Denis Coulombier stepped in. He argued that the February break was a textbook example of what is known as an 'amplifying event' — one that raises the rate at which a disease spreads to a new level.

If there were plans to introduce measures, now was the time.

Then Anders Tegnell replied: there was no need.

The Frenchman looked at the Swede across the table in astonishment.

Tegnell said that, so far, no secondary cases had been identified in Sweden — no individuals who'd picked up the virus from someone inside the country. There was thus no community transmission in Sweden at this point.

Coulombier felt a mounting frustration. That was no way to think. When dealing with a completely new virus, you couldn't ask for perfect data before making decisions. You had to rely on your judgement and the guesses of other experts.

Anders Tegnell's actions were surprising. In epidemiological circles, he was known as the man who'd mass-vaccinated the entire Swedish population against the swine flu in 2009–10. No other country had vaccinated such a large part of its population.

In hindsight, it had turned out to be an overreaction. The flu was mild and soon forgotten. Instead, hundreds of children and young people suffered from narcolepsy as a result of the vaccine.

Now — eleven years later — it appeared that Anders Tegnell was acting in the completely opposite way.

What had happened?

Part I

The patriarch

The new year was only a few days old when a white-haired Swedish state pensioner sat down in front of his computer to check what new diseases might be spreading around the world. Perhaps the plague in Madagascar? Meningitis on Zanzibar? A stomach bug in the US? There was always something exciting going on.

Johan Giesecke was like a retired marine officer following the movements of the US Navy on MarineTraffic with great interest, or like a pilot watching his old planes on Flightradar24.

The old epidemiologist's favourite site was ProMED, a database sprung out of the early internet. There, doctors, veterinarians — indeed, pretty much anyone in the pathogen business — could post early indications and unofficial suspicions that a new contagion was brewing.

Every day there were a dozen or so new posts. In other words, only a fraction of these leads ever developed into epidemics, or pandemics, for that matter. But on here, you'd been able to read about both SARS and MERS in the early days — diseases first appearing in 2003 and 2012 respectively, and caused by entirely new coronaviruses.

Johan Giesecke looked at the screen of his MacBook Air. With age, the skin around his eyebrows had grown increasingly heavy. His eyes, formerly so bright, looked more and more like two diagonal slits.

On this day, he was reading about a new Chinese coronavirus.

Oh well, he thought.

For an epidemiologist, a new virus out of China was a bit like a new murder in Mexico. Serious, sure, but nothing that sparked thoughts other than a reminder of what the world looked like.

He'd seen this before.

Many doctors had been forced into the profession by their parents. We'll meet some of them in this book. For Johan Giesecke, it was the other way around. When he came home one day and said that he wanted to study medicine, his father replied: 'Why?'

'I want to work with people.'

'But do you have to work with sick people?'

His father's name was Curt-Steffan Giesecke, and he was one of Sweden's most powerful people. For twelve years in the 1960s and 1970s, he'd been CEO of the Swedish Employers Association — a position that came with power over millions of workers' salaries, and over thousands of companies' competitiveness.

Curt-Steffan dreamt that his son would one day be the head of one of the crown jewels of Swedish trade: Ericsson, SKF, Sandvik, Astra, SCA, or Volvo. Not that he'd be taking old ladies' temperature and listening to the pulse of geriatrics, or whatever it was that doctors spent their time doing.

Initially, Johan Giesecke followed the trajectory his father had thought out for him, studying engineering and physics at the Royal Institute of Technology in Stockholm. But one day he changed his mind.

And so Giesecke became a doctor. Then he married a doctor. And his three children grew up to become doctors.

Johan Giesecke himself used to say that having so many doctors in the family was idiotic. It would have been more practical if his children had become something else. A car mechanic, a lawyer, and an electrician would have been perfect. And perhaps their conversations at home would have been a little more exciting if his wife had been a literary critic.

In any case, the doctor Johan Giesecke eventually became — despite Curt-Steffan's objections — did contain elements of the engineer and business executive his father had envisioned. The books he wrote were full of equations — if perhaps not as advanced as the ones in the books at the Royal Institute of Technology — and he helped build the European Centre for Disease Prevention and Control, in Solna, as its first chief scientist.

That was a long time ago. Now he was 70 years old and should really have been spending his time at Skärfsta — his manor south of Stockholm, which had once belonged to the famous author Elsa Beskow — raising his sheep, or perhaps sending corrections and letters to the editor to one of the magazines he subscribed to. There was always someone misspelling ectopic pregnancy.

But the virus he was reading about on ProMED this morning would change everything. And not just for Johan Giesecke.

An unclear pneumonia

January of 2020 was a mild month. No snow had settled over the Swedish capital. So when Anders Tegnell arrived in Stockholm by train, he could hop on his old, blue, single-speed bike — the one he always kept locked up outside the Central Station — and pedal north along Vasagatan, across the Norra Bantorget square, and up the gentle but extended incline toward Solna.

Most people cycling in Stockholm wore a helmet. But not the 63-year-old doctor with a physiognomy like a map of Chile, who, sporting a brown jacket and with AirPods in his ears, pedalled through the twin skyscrapers about to be finished at the top of Torsgatan.

When people asked Anders Tegnell why he didn't wear a helmet, he'd say pretty much the same thing as any other grown Swede would: really, it was 'careless' of him, 'bad', and he 'actually did have a helmet at home'.

Once he had passed the towers, he was almost there. The tall buildings formed a portal into the area that was home to Sweden's medical elite. Here was the Karolinska Institute, biomedical startups vying for space, and a newly built colossus of a hospital called New Karolinska, at the time best known for gobbling up tax funds for more than a decade.

The issues troubling Swedish healthcare were well known. Sweden had the lowest number of available hospital beds per capita of all the countries in the EU, and it was worst in Stockholm. A few miles away, on Södermalm, the Södersjukhuset hospital had been forced to go into a state of heightened preparedness a few days earlier — for the fourth time in two years.

The cause of the chaos varied depending on who you asked. Had there been too much privatisation? Too little? Was the organisation lacking? Was it the new digital health centres that were draining the healthcare system of its resources? Was it all because of the rapidly growing and ageing population?

A few hundred yards past the New Karolinska Hospital, Tegnell turned left, and then left again.

On Nobels väg 18, three five-storey buildings in red brick formed an incomplete square. In place of the side missing to complete the geometric shape, three flagpoles signalled that something official went on in the area. From the middle pole hung a shabby, faded flag with the Swedish Public Health Agency's logo: three intersecting hearts under a royal crown. The idea was for the heart shapes to signal 'life, water, and environment', and the yellow colour of the crown to radiate strength and endurance. But without that prior knowledge, the logo looked a bit like a carpet beater without a handle, and was so ugly it had attracted the fury of the state herald, the official in charge of the arms of public offices.

During the first few weeks of the year, Anders Tegnell's inbox was filled with messages about various projects that at first glance seemed peculiarly disparate, but which all fell within the agency's curiously broad mission. The emails concerned everything from preparations ahead of a workshop in Saudi Arabia to a project in Somalia and the screening of newborns in Sweden.

That term — 'public health' — was at once both modern and antiquated.

Much of what the roughly 500 employees in those corridors were busy with were economic considerations; they could be calculating whether it would be cost-effective to offer free vaccinations against a certain infectious disease in a particular region, or evaluating how many years of life could be saved by raising awareness of gambling addiction.

This was a rational, modern, and scientific way of dealing with life, health, and death. In short, making a 40-year-old quit smoking was much cheaper — and more merciful — than surgically removing a tumour from his lungs 15 years later.

This was a science that worshipped metrics and evidence, and measured its victories in increased life expectancy and experienced quality of life. Most of all, it was founded on a belief that humans are malleable creatures, in full alignment with modern terms such as 'nudging' and behavioural economics. If you read the agency's appropriation directions, you might easily gain the impression that its task was to create sober, sporty, and unbiased citizens with a high work attendance.

At the same time, the very notion of a 'public' that could be brought to do anything as a group was somewhat anachronistic: social equality had declined; for decades, there had been such high levels of immigration that, by now, one in every five Swedes had been born outside Sweden; and more than half a million people had signed up for private health insurance.

The social contract upon which public health policy rested — and which compelled Swedes to get vaccinated out of solidarity when the local health centre called, to collectively fund the healthcare system, and to patiently put up with its wait times — was under renegotiation.

When Anders Tegnell stepped into the agency's offices for the first time after the Christmas holiday, he was aware of 'an unclear pneumonia' discovered in the Chinese city of Wuhan. He'd received an email about the mysterious disease while in Spain with his wife and grown children.

When he read the email, he'd reacted in about the same way as Johan Giesecke.

This looked like just another little outbreak that the Chinese could handle.

Chinese whispers

Anders Tegnell wasn't alone in his assessment that the Chinese had the virus under control. On 14 January, the World Health Organization (WHO) confirmed that, as yet, there was no proof the new virus could spread from one person to another.

The problem was that this information came from the Chinese authorities. And for a person in charge of a nation's infectious-disease control, being an expert in viruses and bacteria wasn't really enough. You also needed an understanding of Chinese politics and culture.

After all, that was usually where it started. Almost all the influenza epidemics for which scientists had managed to trace the origins — from the first recorded outbreak in 1888, to the Hong Kong flu in 1968 — had started in China.

It was an ill-fated combination: the country spitting out new viruses each year was also run by a shady dictatorship.

Over the past few years, the situation had grown even more complicated. The outside world's guessing was thwarted by the deteriorating relations between China and the West. Since Xi Jinping had come to power in 2013, China's totalitarian leanings had grown more pronounced. Foreign journalists were finding it harder and harder to work in the country. And because China's economic power was growing each year, the country could now afford to ignore the opinions of the outside world.

Since the Obama years, the Americans had been running a program called 'Predict', which allowed the US Centers for Disease Control and Prevention to place medical observers in locations around China. But after Donald Trump was elected president in 2016, the system fell into decay. Observers who left were never replaced. The last American epidemiologist left the country in 2019.

When reports of a new, mysterious disease began to spread among the world's governments and infectious-disease agencies, the assessments that were made weren't just medical and epidemiological. They were also Kremlinological analyses of what was really happening inside the country.

The suspicion was most evident among China's neighbouring countries. As early as 21 January, Taiwan began to advise against travelling to China. A few days later, this was followed by cancelled flights to the entire country, quarantine for arriving travellers, and an export ban on protective equipment. Similar measures were soon introduced in South Korea.

Around the world, there were signals that the situation was worse than what was being indicated by official statements from China. Companies in the US making protective equipment received gigantic orders from Chinese clients. Reports circulated that hospitals inside China were advising their employees to self-isolate.

Anders Tegnell had a fairly positive view of China. His understanding of the country was that they'd got their act together significantly since the SARS epidemic of 2003. They reported new cases more promptly, and no longer tried to hide epidemics at all costs. Apparently, they had changed tactics.

Moreover, he trusted the global infrastructure that had been built up. Partly because it was the only one there was, and partly because it usually worked well: each country reported its cases, and the WHO acted like a hub, disseminating information to its member states.

To the media, Tegnell said there was no need for Swedes to avoid travelling to China. Not even to affected areas of the country.

The world was prepared, he thought.

What the world didn't know was that, for several weeks, the Chinese authorities had been lying both to their own citizens and to the outside world. A number of doctors who had tried to sound the alarm about the new virus were being investigated by the police. One of them — the eye doctor Li Wenliang — was forced to sign a document in which he promised not to continue his warnings.

Much later, the news agency AP would unearth official documents showing that the regime had known since the middle of January that the situation was much more serious than it claimed.

On 20 January, the Chinese finally admitted that the virus could spread through person-to-person transmission. At the same time, information came in that healthcare workers in the country had been infected.

Transmission within the healthcare system was a classic warning sign. It was the kind of thing you'd see in connection with outbreaks of influenza, measles, or other particularly contagious diseases. It could indicate that isolation-and-control measures had been implemented too late and that there were gaps.

Most countries still chose to hold off on introducing restrictive measures. Both the British Cabinet Office's crisis response group 'COBRA' and the German Robert Koch Institute assessed the level of danger was low.

After all, this wasn't the first time they had received warnings of a dangerous virus out of China. Not even the US, where the authorities had access to the most comprehensive intelligence, issued more than a recommendation to check the temperature of travellers from Wuhan.

On 24 January, Anders Tegnell said to the public broadcaster Sweden's Radio that Swedes had no reason to be concerned.

Desk doctors

In 1662, the British entrepreneur John Graunt published a book with the convoluted title *Natural and Political Observations Made Upon the Bills of Mortality*.

In his book, Graunt analysed the mortality statistics that the Church of England had been keeping for 50 years. Graunt wasn't the only one interested in the numbers. Propertied people in London liked to buy the statistics, which were printed once a week. In this way, they could discover early on if the plague was spreading in the slums, pack up their belongings, and temporarily move outside the city.

But what Graunt did was to go back in history. He collated thousands of old documents, many of them hard to decipher, and sketched out mortality patterns: when and how many had people died, and of what?

Suddenly, a lot became clear. There were years when the plague completely vanished, and years when it swept through the population. In 1625, it had killed 46,000 people — 38,000 more than all other causes of death combined.

But it wasn't just the ebb and flow of the plague that emerged from the numbers. What Graunt further discovered was a mortality rate that remained consistent during years without epidemics. There was an 'expected' number of deaths among the population — and when the plague raged you could subtract that number from the total death toll to find out how severe the epidemic was.

It was as though it was possible to be a doctor without even going near a patient.

Around this time, the theories held by physicians about the plague assumed there was a 'miasma', a kind of gas, influenced by the positions of the planets, that emanated out of the ground and infected people. That is why many doctors wore large 'beaks' filled with dried flowers, honey, and herbs when they went to see their patients. The plague doctors' dress became a cultural icon — even today, their bird-like costume can be seen at carnivals and on theatre stages — but the face masks of the day didn't offer any protection.

Using Graunt's tables, it was possible to guess a lot of things about how the plague spread, how fast it arose, and when it would go away again. But the doctors of the time do not appear to have noticed what Graunt was up to. The belief in astrological causes lived on.

There are no signs that the contemporaneous medical sciences took Graunt's statistical conclusions to heart. Possibly his theories may have gained a stronger hold among decision-makers of the time. At any rate, his book sold well enough for several editions to be printed in the seventeenth century.

The last big plague epidemic in London occurred in 1665. But what role the statistical gains may have played remains unclear; a lot happened in these years. Stricter quarantine rules were imposed, the rat population changed, and more houses were built of stone rather than of wood, separating the infectious rats from the humans.

Perhaps John Graunt's theories were of no significance whatsoever to the healing arts. But long before anyone had ever seen a virus through a microscope, long before anyone even knew it was viruses or bacteria that caused common sicknesses, he took the initial steps in the science now known as epidemiology.

Three and a half centuries after Graunt compiled his death tables, epidemiology engaged tens of thousands of people across the world: statisticians, doctors, mathematicians, programmers.

But somehow it remained the same as in the seventeenth century: this was a discipline concerned with patterns and large-scale correlation, not individual cases.

Thinking in terms of 'populations', as epidemiologists liked to call their groups of people, didn't come naturally to all doctors. Perhaps they once took up medicine for idealistic reasons. To save lives. To care for people.

And for most of medical history, doctors had been in the business of diagnosing individuals. But for the epidemiologist, a single death was just that — a single death — and meaningful conclusions could only be drawn if there were more.

Johan Giesecke liked to say that both kinds were needed. There was a need for doctors who looked after patients, and there was a need for doctors like him: the kind he called 'desk doctors'.

Desk doctors disassembled patients into their quantifiable constituent parts — sex, age, location, profession, weight, height — to find a type of information impossible to discover at an individual level. Is exposure to asbestos dangerous? Is cervical cancer contagious?

Infectious diseases weren't all they cared about. Any puzzle piece that could help people live longer and healthier lives was of interest.

But epidemiology wasn't just about finding patterns and correlations in different populations. It was also a science about what to do with that information once you had it.

It's one thing to treat a single patient. It's quite another to treat a whole population. With these new tools came a number of thorny moral and ethical — political — problems.

The first one cropped up roughly a hundred years after John Graunt had taken the first step in epidemiology.

The casino

Every day, the people walking the Earth in the eighteenth century ran a considerable risk of catching the plague, tuberculosis, cholera, or one of the other diseases moving invisibly through the world's populations.

Perhaps the most feared disease was smallpox. It had already tormented humanity for thousands of years. As the Spaniards conquered Mexico around 1520, they unknowingly brought it with them, causing 18 million Mexicans — out of a population of 25 million — to succumb almost immediately. Over the century that followed, smallpox continued to kill off the indigenous Mexican population, until only 1.6 million remained.

Across the world, the disease could decimate a population. An outbreak in Iceland in 1707 killed 18,000 out of a population of 50,000.

It wasn't just the high death rate that frightened people. The symptoms were excruciating, and the course of the disease was slow. 'The entire body from head to foot is encrusted with innumerable pustules flowing into each other and burning like fire … a brown crust finally covers the entire body and face, and out of its fissures a stinking, rotten pus emerges, which has often dissolved the flesh down to the bone: one no longer sees a human in the face of the sick,' wrote the Swedish physician Eberhard Zacharias Munck af Rosenschöld.

But in the eighteenth century, the situation in Europe changed. Suddenly, there was an alternative to passively awaiting epidemics. Suddenly, it was possible to buy something that could be likened to a lottery ticket.

Around this time in England, there was a new practice of scratching secretions or pus from smallpox pustules into the skin of healthy people. It was a dangerous procedure. Many died from the inoculation itself, but most survived. And if they did, they appeared to have a strong protection against smallpox.

Many renowned Enlightenment philosophers endorsed these modern methods. The most famous of them, Voltaire, had been to England and witnessed it himself.

Others questioned whether such a risk could even be taken: there was insufficient information about the deadliness of the disease and the effects of immunisation.

In the years 1750–70, the issue was hotly debated all over Europe.

Buy the lottery ticket or not?

This was when epidemiology stepped into uncharted territory. And it started as a bit of a side project, a footnote in the career of one of the eighteenth century's most influential scientists.

Daniel Bernoulli came from a family of prominent mathematicians — and wanted to become one himself. But, initially, Bernoulli's father opposed his chosen profession. It simply didn't pay well. Daniel's father, Johann Bernoulli, was one of the leading mathematicians of his time, and constantly complained about his low salary. After all, this was almost three centuries before the hedge funds of the world discovered that it's possible to trade stocks using algorithms, and started paying handsomely for any form of mathematical talent.

But even in those days, what led to riches was trade and finance. The Bernoulli family had once been wealthy traders, and Daniel's father wanted him to make it prosperous once more.

Mathematics most certainly wasn't the way. Daniel's grandfather had grown rich trading spices, and something along those lines was the plan for the talented Daniel Bernoulli.

But Daniel wasn't feeling it.

Slowly, his father softened. At first, he let his son study medicine as a kind of compromise. But, eventually, he started teaching him mathematics.

Daniel Bernoulli never married, never had children. Instead, he mass-produced mathematical proofs, technical innovations, and solutions to problems. The basics of today's aeroplane wings and combustion engines were born inside his brain.

Today, Bernoulli's name adorns lecture halls at institutions in everything from mathematics and economics to behavioural science and marine technology.

He is less well known in the medical sciences. But it was when he applied his mathematical knowledge to the smallpox dilemma that something revolutionary happened.

Daniel Bernoulli started playing around with some tables compiled by Edmond Halley — the guy with the comet — a hundred years earlier. The tables showed the number of children and young adults who had died in a Polish city in the seventeenth century.

First, Bernoulli made some assumptions: that the risk of catching smallpox was the same across all ages, that the mortality rate was 12.5 per cent, and that it didn't vary by age.

Then he set up an equation to calculate what proportion of the population in each age group had never had smallpox — and then a second equation that showed how many lives would have been saved if the disease had never existed.

The results were as clear as day. If every person in the Polish town had undergone immunisation, life expectancy would have increased by more than three years.

He realised that figure was difficult for people to grasp, however. So he expressed it another way: out of 1,300 newborns, 565 would live until they were at least 25 years old if nothing was done. But if smallpox was eradicated, 644 would live to that same age.

It was a matter of 79 human lives.

Here were two ways of looking at the same thing. But by expressing it in the number of children who would will survive, 'we bestow', in Bernoulli's words, 'the advantage directly and entirely on those who are saved'.

It no doubt sounded better.

He had yet another way of expressing this value — one that would appeal to the social elite of the era: by adopting universal inoculation against smallpox, 'France would annually gain 25,000 people, all useful to the State'.

Bernoulli also saw the risks involved in the scratching. But his calculations showed that the benefits far outweighed the costs.

This was a lottery ticket that everyone should buy.

Not only that. This was a lottery ticket that the state should buy for all its citizens.

The science known as epidemiology is sometimes described as the study of the causes and spread of diseases. Who gets sick and from what?

What that description leaves out is that epidemiologists can sometimes *decide* who gets sick and why.

Daniel Bernoulli was willing to accept a few people dying of immunisation against smallpox in order to save many more from dying of smallpox. In the same way, today's epidemiologists, public-health experts, and politicians weigh the risks against the benefits for everything from vaccination programs to the use of pharmaceuticals and chlorination of our drinking water.

Daniel Bernoulli's calculation didn't just prove the value of vaccinating a population.

Once he had planted the seed for modern ways of thinking about disease and epidemics, it wasn't just the modern science of epidemiology and public health that sprouted, but also an ethical debate that has remained strikingly unchanged.

It was Bernoulli's nemesis, the French mathematician and physician Jean le Rond d'Alembert, who put his finger on the issue.

Imagine another disease, d'Alembert explained — with other odds. As fictive as it is improbable, you can immunise yourself against it. And a person who survives the procedure is guaranteed to live until the age of 100. The problem is that one in five people die from the immunisation.

According to Bernoulli's way of thinking, d'Alembert argued, it would be right for the state to advocate mass immunisation even when the risks were that high. But few citizens — perhaps none — would be so brave or stupid as to accept these odds.

D'Alembert was not an opponent of immunisation in general. On the contrary, he seemed to think the smallpox ticket in particular was a sensible one to buy. But it was far from as simple as Daniel Bernoulli or Voltaire would have you think.

The individual's calculation was not the same as that of the state. From the perspective of a social engineer, the population might look like poker chips in a giant casino.

But this wasn't hydrodynamics, trigonometry, probability theory, or any of the other things that Daniel Bernoulli had worked on. There was an ethical dimension to the combating of infectious diseases that you couldn't get away from.

There was a difference between being the gambler and being the stake. A human being only has one life — the state has millions.

And with that, the battle lines were drawn.

Giesecke's boy

If there was one person who could step into Daniel Bernoulli's casino and calculate the odds without any anxiety, it was the man who in the spring of 2020 held the somewhat archaic title of state epidemiologist of Sweden.

To Anders Tegnell, there were two ways of mentally approaching his job: either you began to fret, or you tuned out.

Tegnell was the kind who tuned out.

That's how he described himself. And surely it said something about his person that the only words spoken against him were ones he spoke of himself.

Those who had studied and worked with Tegnell said that he was prudent, controlled, and unaffected by pressure and stress. Those who'd worked under him said that he was a rather typical manager at a Swedish government agency, the kind who put his own coffee mug in the dishwasher.

Tegnell himself said that he was a bit square. When describing himself, he was even known to make squares in the air with his hands.

Back in the day when he saw patients, he hadn't really clicked with those who worried and wanted their diagnoses couched in lots of fluff and sympathy. He worked best with patients who preferred clear and unambiguous messages.

Tegnell thought the Swedish people were like the former type of patient: they were fearful, bad at managing risk.

Tegnell himself had lived all over, both in Sweden and the world — in Ethiopia, Östersund, Laos, the US, Lund — and thought himself able to see his home country from the outside a bit. His theory about the reason for the Swedish people's fearfulness was that they had lived in peace for such a long time.

Now they seemed worried about that new Chinese virus.

* * *

But we are getting ahead of ourselves. The story of how Anders Tegnell ended up at the Public Health Agency of Sweden began one day in the late 1990s. That was when he first met Johan Giesecke.

At the time, Giesecke was Sweden's state epidemiologist, and a group of infectious-disease doctors from all over the country had come to Stockholm for a meeting. Exactly what was discussed at the meeting has fallen into oblivion, but Johan Giesecke immediately noticed the gangly man at the far end of the table, still with a splash of colour on his face after a sojourn in Laos.

Then Tegnell opened his mouth to speak.

Wow, Giesecke thought when he heard his quaint dialect. *This kid is completely apolitical.*

To Johan Giesecke, 'apolitical' was the finest thing a person could be. He liked it when people spoke their mind and did what they were supposed to, without reflecting too much on what was expedient or politically viable at the time.

Like many men of his generation, Johan Giesecke had a habit of telling the same stories over and over, as though the written language had not yet been invented and the only way to keep the anecdotes alive was to pass them down orally to as many people as possible like some ancient rhapsode.

One of Giesecke's favourite stories was about Jan Eliasson, the Swedish top diplomat who later became both foreign minister and deputy secretary-general of the United Nations, and whose self-absorption inspired the nickname '*Jag* Eliasson' (Swedish for 'I, Eliasson') in the corridors of the Ministry for Foreign Affairs.

The story had been adapted a little over the years, but essentially went like this: Jan Eliasson had received news of an impending crisis. Perhaps a pandemic, perhaps one of the countless scandals exposed within the UN system over the years.

'This isn't good,' Eliasson said. 'This isn't good for me.'

At which his colleagues stared at their boss. He stared back, and added: 'And not for the UN, of course.' (Many years later, the US political satire TV series *Veep* would be based on the same kind of narcissism.)

Another of Giesecke's anecdotes was about a member of the Swedish parliament who, at some point in the 1960s, had suggested that all spirits sold at the government-owned monopoly liquor store should be enriched with thiamine, or vitamin B_1. The reason was that many alcoholics were suffering from diseases that could be attributed to a thiamine deficiency.

It was actually a good idea. Had Giesecke been a member of parliament, he would have voted for it.

But the proposal failed. Of course. It had sent the 'wrong signals', or something along those lines.

What was right from a medical perspective — what was right from a public health perspective — wasn't always right from a political perspective. This was an insight striking many of the doctors who'd risen to high positions in the borderland between medicine and politics.

Him, I'll have, Giesecke thought at his first meeting with Anders Tegnell. *He's going to work in Stockholm.*

Besides, he mused, the young man had just returned from Laos. He ought to be moveable.

At this time, Johan Giesecke's recruitment process was more similar to the way things might have worked in a family-run business than at a Swedish government agency: he'd find a person — typically a man — hire him, and only then begin to come up with assignments for him.

Tegnell did not object to Giesecke's plans for him. He took the job, but never moved to Stockholm. He chose to stay in Linköping, where he'd moved into his childhood home with his wife.

Giesecke became his mentor. And Tegnell became Giesecke's boy. That's what he called him: his boy.

Giesecke helped his protégé finish a thesis on the risks of infection associated with heart surgery — and eventually it so happened that Anders Tegnell became the state epidemiologist of Sweden.

That was in 2013, almost two decades after their first meeting in Stockholm.

So when all of Sweden — indeed, large parts of the world — were struck by how unmoved, how unwavering Anders Tegnell was during the coronavirus pandemic, it wasn't so strange after all.

That's why he'd been chosen.

That's why he was Giesecke's boy.

The war

Being a desk doctor could be quite exciting.

Once, a long time ago — in 1998, to be exact — Johan Giesecke had got his hands on three different lists. These were registers of blood donors, patients who'd received a blood transfusion, and individuals infected with HIV in Sweden. Giesecke had got them from a chief physician in Stockholm.

With the help of some data magic, he and a colleague managed to sift out 100 individuals who may have been infected with HIV. The reason was that they'd received blood just before 1985, the year when all propsective blood donors had to undertake an HIV test.

But the National Board of Health and Welfare stopped the project. In a letter to Giesecke, the agency wrote that the project was 'very dubious from both a legal and an ethical standpoint'.

They wrote about it in the papers and everything. It left a little scar.

To be a desk doctor, you didn't just need to know mathematics and medicine. You also needed to navigate through a thicket of law, ethics, and politics.

And Giesecke made a comeback. A few years later, he'd learnt his lesson. This time, he started with a list of 350 patients who had recently been infected with HIV. After conversations with each of them, he identified 550 people who might have been infected by the original 350. In the end, he found another 50 cases of infection.

These were 50 human beings who could now receive treatment. Fifty human lives. And it was all above board.

When Johan Giesecke spoke about the pandemics he'd experienced, he sounded at times like an old soldier, inked and scarred, spinning yarns about his adventurous life for his grandchildren.

HIV, SARS, swine flu, avian flu. As though he carried medals from each war on his chest.

HIV had been the worst.

Pandemics were like wars in more ways than one. It wasn't just a question of *how* to fight — but *whether* to fight.

It was easy to remember the times when politicians and infectious-disease experts had waited too long to act, like during the HIV epidemic. But history also contained examples of when politicians and epidemiologists had overreacted.

The classic example was the 1976 swine flu in the US. The Americans believed that a new, deadly pandemic was on the rise. They rushed out a vaccine and prepared for mass vaccinations. President Gerald Ford and his wife each got the shot in front of the TV cameras to encourage their citizens to do the same.

Pretty soon, side effects began to be reported. A few of those who'd received the vaccine appeared to be afflicted with Guillain-Barré syndrome — a disease paralysing the patient's arms and legs.

The vaccination campaign was paused pending an investigation into these cases. And it was never resumed. What's more, the flu turned out to be much milder than the experts had predicted.

The US government was forced to pay large amounts in damages to those afflicted — even though no one could say with certainty that the vaccine had caused the disorder.

Yet the biggest damage wasn't financial. The incident sparked a mistrust between citizens and government agencies that eventually led to the anti-vax movement. Suddenly, people stopped vaccinating their children against measles and polio.

The scars from 1976 were also one of the reasons why it took so long for the authorities to act on HIV.

The swine flu in the 1970s was the Vietnam War of epidemiology.

Johan Giesecke and Anders Tegnell had also fought a needless war, each from their corner. This, too, was against a swine flu that turned out to be milder than anyone thought.

We'll soon return to that story.

The first case

On 24 January 2020 — the same day that Anders Tegnell assured the Swedish people that there was no need to worry about the new virus — a young woman returned home to Jönköping, Sweden. She had been on a visit to Wuhan, China, but was feeling well.

By this time, a couple of hundred Chinese had fallen ill after being infected with the novel coronavirus. Out of them, 25 had died.

At least, that's what the Chinese were reporting to the WHO. What was actually going on inside the country no one knew with certainty. The US Centers for Disease Control and Prevention, the CDC, had offered to send personnel to China, but the Chinese government hadn't responded to the offer.

What the outside world did know was that the Chinese authorities had isolated the 11 million inhabitants of Wuhan from the rest of China. But while it was no longer possible to fly from Wuhan to Beijing, people could still travel from Wuhan to London, New York, Milan, or Stockholm.

Slowly, the virus began to seep out into the world.

Four days after returning home, the woman in Jönköping developed a bit of a cough. Two days later — on 30 January — she contacted the healthcare services. It turned out that she was infected with the coronavirus. She was isolated at Ryhov County Hospital in Jönköping. Sweden had its first case. It was one of roughly 150 cases discovered outside China.

A week earlier, the director-general of the Swedish Public Health Agency, Johan Carlson, had ordered that the coronavirus be 'treated as a special event within the agency where special procedures are activated'. Now the bureaucratic machinery began to be cranked up with greater force. On 3 February, the agency's leadership decided that a special crisis-management organisation be set up. Three days later, Carlson travelled to the Swedish parliament to inform the Committee on Health and Welfare about the new virus.

* * *

Even though the foundation was now being laid for stronger measures, Anders Tegnell stuck to his opinion that the risk of transmission in Sweden was low — indeed, 'very low', according to his agency's official risk assessment.

And during the weeks to come, the virus appeared to be spreading slowly. By Thursday 13 February, the WHO had only racked up 447 cases in 24 countries outside China.

What's more, within China the spread of the virus appeared to have stalled. For two weeks, the reported number of new cases had hovered between 2,000 and 4,000 per day, and now it seemed as though the increase was subsiding a little.

But that Thursday, new information emerged out of China. The authorities had changed their definition of what counted as a case. Now, they suddenly had 15,000 new cases — in one day.

It began to collectively dawn on the world that the initial information from the Chinese had not been worth much. What's more, the week prior, Li Wenliang — the Chinese doctor who had been punished for his warnings — had passed away after being infected with the new virus.

Fear began to spread. From 20 February, the value of the world's public companies fell with each passing day. Initially, the situation was interpreted as a supply crisis. Because China had become the whole world's factory, many believed there would soon be a shortage of everything from car parts to circuit boards and mobile phones. But soon panic spread to more countries. Companies across all industries were dragged down in the fall.

The world's stock markets had decided a crisis was looming — but its epidemiologists were still hesitant.

The number of cases grew and grew and grew.

Was it time to act? To go to war?

Thus far, the mystery about the new virus had moved in the borderlands between medicine and Chinese Kremlinology. But in the space of just a few weeks, the world had found out that the virus spread through person-to-person transmission, that it was quite contagious, and that it had begun to spread outside China.

And it was now that it turned into a mathematical problem.

The letter R

Ronald Ross fell in love with mathematics late in life.

Mathematical proofs were like works of art. And endless sequences of numbers were like musical compositions, piano sonatas.

But it was too late for mathematics. Much too late. What was he — a British doctor — going to do with mathematics? He felt like a married man drawn to another woman.

Becoming a doctor hadn't even been his decision. Like many men before him and after, he was coerced into studying medicine by his father. Ronald himself had dreamt of becoming an author, a poet, perhaps a musician. He didn't even pass all the elements of his medical degree.

Though perhaps Daddy Ross deserves some small recognition, as Ronald did pretty okay as a doctor after all. When the Nobel Prize in Medicine was awarded in 1902 — for just the second time ever — it was given to Ronald Ross for his work on malaria.

Malaria was a disease that interested the Brits, who for the past couple of centuries had made it their national pastime to colonise faraway countries. When British soldiers and officials served in tropical and subtropical areas, many of them came down with fever and chills, combined with nausea, vomiting, and muscle aches. The symptoms were similar to the flu, in other words, but this disease was much worse.

Ross received the Nobel Prize for showing how malaria spread in humans, for the discovery that mosquitoes carried the infection from one human to another with their bites. And the number of mosquitoes, in turn, depended on the number of water repositories in the vicinity. By removing water tanks from military bases, for example, the disease could be curbed.

Ross should probably have shared the prize with his mentor, Patrick Manson, who was the first to suspect that mosquitoes transmitted the disease. Before that, the world's doctors had been guessing blindly. The word malaria comes from the Italian *mala aria*

— bad air — which was one of the hypotheses about the cause of the disease in the Middle Ages.

Ross didn't even tell Manson that he'd been given the prize. It was an interesting strategy, but keeping a Nobel Prize secret turned out to be difficult. Manson eventually read about it in the papers, which led to a long enmity between the two doctors.

The malaria theory didn't just land Ronald Ross a Nobel Prize and an indignant mentor. It also gave him an opportunity to deepen his love for mathematics.

He wondered: might it be possible to eradicate malaria without killing every mosquito on Earth?

He started writing out equations. Suppose there was one individual infected with malaria in a village of 1,000 people. In order for the disease to spread, a mosquito would have to find the infected individual specifically.

Ross assumed that only one in every four mosquitoes managed to bite someone. There would thus have to be 4,000 mosquitoes for one to start carrying the disease.

But that wasn't enough. It takes some time for the malaria parasite to reproduce inside the mosquito, and during that time the insect could die.

He kept on writing his equations. Solving and making assumptions. Finally, he came to the conclusion that it would require 48,000 mosquitoes to generate a single additional infection in his fictitious village.

There was thus a critical threshold. If the number of mosquitoes fell below it, the disease could no longer spread.

In true mathematical spirit, he called his insight the 'mosquito theorem'.

* * *

In the years following the Second World War, malaria doctors began to suspect that very tiny changes were needed for an epidemic to escalate.

A model developed as early as 1927 by the scientists William Ogilvy Kermack and Anderson Gray McKendrick — yes, they too were British — came to be of great significance. It was called the 'SIR model', and divided populations into three groups: susceptible, infected, and recovered.

As epidemics spread, people flowed eastward through the equation. From S to I to R.

In London, the scientist George MacDonald now began to list factors that could affect the rate at which a disease spread. Take a regular cold, for example. How much it spreads doesn't just depend on the cold virus itself. Its infectivity also depends on the infected individual's living situation, how many people they encounter on the Metro on their way to work, how many they work with, how long they stay sick, how they behave during that time.

MacDonald studied malaria, which made things even more complicated. A simple detail like the number of pigs in a village could affect the spread of infection, as every time a mosquito chose to make a pig its victim, a human being was spared.

MacDonald condensed all this information into what he called the reproduction number.

In the scientific literature produced by epidemiologists today, the number is usually represented as R_0 (pronounced as 'Reff' or 'R-naught', depending on what country you're in). This signifies the expected number of people who will be infected by each sick person if everyone else is susceptible to infection. It differs from the effective reproduction number, which changes as people become infected, recover, or get vaccinated.

But in essence, it's the same concept that MacDonald came up with: if the value of R is lower than 1, it means that each infected individual will transmit the disease to fewer than one other person. In such a situation, an epidemic can never take off.

But a value well above 1 is like the spark that ignites the flame.

Let's say the value of R_0 is 4. If so, the first person will infect four others. Those four, in turn, will infect another four — each. And so on.

Self-confidence soared high when the World Health Organization, the WHO, was formed in 1948. Now malaria was finally going to be eradicated. They had the money, the equations — and the chemicals. The discovery of dichlorodiphenyltrichloroethane — also known as DDT — seemed a powerful weapon against the mosquitoes transmitting the malaria parasite. Combined with an ambitious program for treatment, monitoring, and isolation of sick patients, it would be possible to break the chain through which the infection spread between mosquitoes and people.

But it turned out to be harder than they'd thought.

A few years earlier, MacDonald had been out in the field. On the island of Ceylon, now Sri Lanka, he'd witnessed the aftermath of a malaria epidemic that claimed the lives of 80,000 people. As he went through his data, he drew the conclusion that the reproduction number was somewhere around 10.

Such high R numbers were bad news for the malaria warriors. But it was about to get worse. In his 2012 book *Spillover*, the author David Quammen recounts what happened when MacDonald continued his calculations. MacDonald imagined one single malaria-infected individual evading diagnosis and remaining infectious for days. It wasn't unreasonable to assume that he could be exposed to ten mosquitoes per day.

What reproduction number would this yield?

The answer: 540.

One single malaria-infected individual could infect 540 others.

Game over.

IAt one and the same time MacDonald had invented the reproduction number, and had snuffed out all hope of successfully eradicating malaria.

The fact that he'd chosen the letter R to designate the reproduction number was a bit unfortunate, as that letter was already in use by the SIR model — where it referred to the number of people who had recovered.

But then again, this was a specialised science. R numbers weren't really something ordinary people would ever have to worry about, were they?

* * *

At the Swedish Public Health Agency, it was the Department of Public Health Analysis and Data Management that kept track of infectious outbreaks across the world. This was the department that Anders Tegnell was in charge of.

In turn, the department had seven sub-units. It was the 'unit for analysis' that was responsible for calculating the probability that Sweden would be hit by the new virus.

The head of the unit was Lisa Brouwers. She had long experience of working with complex models. Her doctoral thesis was titled *Microsimulation Models for Disaster Policy Making*, and dealt specifically with simulations of two different kinds of disasters: floods and epidemics.

Brouwers made the assessment that MacDonald's reproduction number couldn't be used to calculate the spread of the novel coronavirus. It wasn't one homogenous outbreak, but multiple local ones.

Instead of R_0, she preferred to use something known as CAR. This was an acronym for 'clinical attack rate', and was a measurement often used in influenza outbreaks. By dividing the number of sick individuals in a population by the total number of people, you could arrive at a percentage reflecting how many were in need of care. This attack rate could also be calculated for different social groups: the elderly, people with co-morbidities, school children, etc.

Its simplicity and clarity made it a useful measurement. As the calculation was based solely on people with symptoms, there was no need to guess how many were infected without displaying any symptoms.

But sitting on the other side of Lake Brunnsviken was a mathematics professor more fond of R numbers. And he came up with entirely different figures for how the virus would strike against Sweden.

The mathematician

Tom Britton usually led a fairly quiet life. Every morning, the fair-haired 55-year-old would get on his bike outside his home on Gärdet in Stockholm. Then he'd pedal his way through the northern parts of town before arriving at an old red-brick building by Lake Brunnsviken.

Surrounded by grand deciduous trees and towered buildings from the early twentieth century, the campus — known as Kräftriket, the 'crayfish kingdom' — might have resembled the grounds of an American ivy league college if it weren't so dilapidated.

Only a small part of Stockholm University had ended up here, about a mile from the rest of campus. Here you would find, among other bits and pieces, the psychology department, the department of Asian studies, and the secretariat for polar research.

The mathematicians resided in Building 6. Inside, Britton usually walked around in jeans and a button-up shirt, sometimes with a baseball cap pushed down over his unruly mathematician's hair. He spent his days punching out code and supervising students writing essays on how to predict National Hockey League results or explain traffic accidents using logistic-regression models.

At the start of February 2020, Britton was busy preparing a workshop on infectious-disease modelling taking place in Luminy, a small town outside Marseille. He had invited mathematicians and statisticians from all over the world, and 50 scientists had RSVPd.

But just a few days before he was due to hop on a plane to France, his computer dinged. One scientist after another wrote to say they couldn't make it. In a short space of time, five of them dropped out.

Their reason was the new virus in China.

Tom Britton found this fascinating. He'd read about the virus before, without making much of it. But the five dropouts piqued his interest. He rearranged the schedule for the workshop a little, adding one more item: a meeting about the Chinese virus.

Then he boarded the plane.

The conference in the little village near the Mediterranean began on 17 February. Forty-five scientists followed the schedule that Britton had laid out. They presented some research findings, talked mathematics, and got to know each other.

It was a conference like any other.

That night, it was time for the session on the new coronavirus. And the first to take the floor was the British professor Julia Gog from Cambridge University: 'I know you're all working on very interesting research projects ...' she began.

She went on to say politely that the participants' projects were all very important. For even theoretical models of unclear practical use contributed to the advancement of science.

Then she said: 'But you have to drop them now.'

This new virus required mobilisation. Over the next six months, she and other scientists with a more practical focus would need all the help they could get to understand how the virus operated.

Tom Britton was all ears.

When Tom Britton was young, people would always ask him if he was going to become a doctor. He was a good student, and both his mother and father were doctors.

He grew so tired of the question that he decided to become anything but a doctor. So when a teacher in upper secondary school suggested he should keep going with mathematics, he latched on to the idea.

There are many kinds of mathematicians in the world, but they could all be placed on a spectrum based on what type of problem they like to solve.

At one end are those who deal with obscure, theoretical stuff: mathematical proofs, theorems, things that may never be of any practical use.

At the other end are those who like to calculate the weather, heat conduction, financial models, insurance premiums — things of clear practical significance to people. They might even be able to explain to someone at a party what it is they do for a living.

Tom Britton thought he fell somewhere around the middle. His research focused on phenomena that could be experienced in the real world — such as social networks or mathematical relations between species, genes, and individuals, or the way diseases spread. But his publications were mostly about the methods behind those calculations. Most of the time, he wasn't calculating R_0 or drawing other conclusions about specific diseases.

His students and doctoral supervisees took a slightly different view of him. They saw — and liked — that he was close to a kind of mathematics that regular people might not be able to grasp, but the usefulness of which they could at least appreciate.

Britton had certainly been guilty of playing to the gallery in his time. In the summer of 2011, when the same man from southern Sweden scored two jackpots with two separate scratch lottery tickets, Britton went on TV4's morning talk show to explain how unlikely that was to happen — the probability was less than one in 160 billion.

He could also be found writing short replies to op-eds when some economist had made an obvious computational error. In 2018, when the Swedish Government Defence Commission wanted to emphasise the growing threat against Sweden by changing the traditional wording that an armed attack on Sweden was 'unlikely' to it 'cannot be ruled out', Britton questioned whether — from a mathematical standpoint — this implied a bigger threat at all.

Many found him funny that way. And if Swedes had been a little more interested in mathematics, perhaps he might even have been a celebrity.

But he wasn't. Not yet.

The fifth pandemic

Johan Giesecke had truly seen this before.

In June 2003, he'd travelled around in a white minivan in the Chinese province of Inner Mongolia on a mission for the WHO.

Every 100 kilometres, he had been stopped by government officials in white spacesuits checking his temperature. Once they had made sure it was below 38 degrees Celsius, he had been allowed to pass.

Everywhere, he and his colleagues had been checked: at the airport, at every hospital they visited, in restaurants, at the hotel.

What would have happened if we'd had a fever? he often wondered.

This was during the SARS epidemic. The four letters in the acronym described the symptoms of the disease: Severe Acute Respiratory Syndrome.

The times, they were a-changing — even back then. A few decades earlier, the disease would have been given an exciting name with a geographical twist, the kind that medical history is full of: the West Nile virus, Ebola, the Asian flu pandemic, the Spanish flu.

Things were more complicated now. The countries of the world weren't too excited about seeing years of brand-building destroyed just because some local happened to eat the wrong bat. And there were others who could be pissed off, too: a Japanese man named Noro once submitted a complaint to the International Committee on Taxonomy of Viruses, asking them to rename the norovirus. There were almost 20,000 Noros in Japan, none of whom was too keen on being associated with a virus also known as the winter vomiting bug.

The WHO eventually drew up some guidelines: avoid names of places, people, and animals. But names describing symptoms are fine.

So, in 2003, the world settled on SARS. But for a long time, the cause of the disease remained unclear: hantavirus? *E. coli*? Typhus?

The regime in Beijing favoured a theory that the deaths were caused by a chlamydia bacterium — probably because it would aim fewer suspicions at the 'wet markets', where everything from snakes and porcupines to beavers and bats were slaughtered onsite.

Eventually, a group of scientists at the University of Hong Kong found the guilty virus. When they saw it with their own eyes in the electron microscope, they noticed that each virus particle was surrounded by little spikes.

Browsing through the archives, they eventually found a match. This was a new member of the coronavirus family. They had been named specifically for the crown — or *corona* — of protein spikes surrounding them.

There were other coronaviruses. Some of them caused common colds in people; others gave rise to hepatitis in mice, or breathing difficulties for turkeys.

But the virus that was spreading in 2003 was different. If a person between the age of 25 and 44 was infected with SARS, the fatality rate was 6 per cent — and it rose with age. The risk of dying was more than 50 per cent for those over the age of 65.

The virus was given the awkward name 'SARS coronavirus' — abbreviated as SARS-CoV — and soon the entire Chinese control apparatus was activated. People suspected of being infected were isolated for two weeks. At one point, 3 million Chinese worked full-time on combating the virus.

When Johan Giesecke returned home, he told Swedish newspapers what he had seen. It was possible to control such an infectious disease, but only with truly draconian methods.

During this time, Canada was also hit by the SARS epidemic. It took the Canadians much longer to get on top of the virus. Sprung out of British democracy, the North American country was on the whole a little more reluctant to lock people up without very good reason.

There was, simply put, a difference between democracies and dictatorships.

Now, 17 years after SARS, the world was learning more and more about another coronavirus. It had been given an even more awkward name — SARS-CoV-2. Just like the previous SARS virus, it caused a potentially severe acute respiratory infection. The WHO named the new illness 'Coronavirus Disease 2019' — or Covid-19.

The virus was apparently not as deadly as the one that caused the first SARS epidemic. But it was more contagious.

As it sent the world spiralling down into what looked like a recession, a tiny sector of the economy blew up. Suddenly, there was a big demand for epidemiologists — even retired ones.

Johan Giesecke was already part of one 'STAG'. The acronym was short for 'Strategic and Technical Advisory Group', and it was one of many advisory panels to the World Health Organization. There were groups for everything from neglected tropical diseases to antibiotic resistance. The group that Giesecke was part of had been formed in 2018, after the Ebola outbreak in Africa, and was known as STAG-IH. The last two letters stood for 'infectious hazards'. The group's task was to offer technical and strategic advice to both the WHO and its member states.

In February 2020, Johan Giesecke's computer started dinging. Soon, he'd have nine different jobs: on one committee here, one advisory role there.

The 70-year-old epidemiologist was back.

This would be his fifth pandemic.

The hypochondriacal Malthusian

Björn Olsen was like an inverted version of one of the figureheads at the Public Health Agency. While the rest of the epidemiological elite in Sweden more or less all descended from academic families, Björn Olsen hailed from a social class many of them had only seen in films or read about in books.

Björn Olsen's parents had been so poor they had been forced to put him in an orphanage when he was six years old. It was at this young age that the foundation was laid for his suspicion of bureaucrats and officials. His conversations with case workers from Social Services over the years were Kafkaesque. He always had to weigh his answers carefully to make sure no sibling got in trouble.

Not many believed Björn Olsen would one day become a chief physician and professor. When he was allowed to graduate from Year Nine, despite incomplete grades, the justification noted that at least he wasn't 'sniffing paint thinner'.

Somehow, Olsen managed to make up for the grades he needed — and, somehow again, got into medical school in Uppsala. But after attending a dissection, he came down with the flu and was completely knocked out for two weeks. He didn't have a phone, because he couldn't afford one, so he couldn't call the university and tell them he was sick.

When he returned, he found that the teachers had given his spot to someone on the waitlist. They had thought he was too soft, that he couldn't handle the sight of a dead person. That he was a weakling.

There was a grain of truth in that assessment. Björn Olsen suffered from a fairly severe form of hypochondria, and believed himself to be afflicted with more or less every disease they learned about in Uppsala. The only time he didn't have to worry was in gynaecology class.

But he had no problem with death. He saw it everywhere, all the time, and one thing he pondered about a lot was how humanity would eventually die out. He was interested in the demographer and economist Thomas Malthus's 200-year-old theories about population explosions leading to mass death, only to be followed by more population explosions.

That alone was pretty rare. Anyone who had ever studied for a Swedish degree in economics had been taught one single fact about the Englishman Malthus: that he was wrong. Technical innovations and more efficient means of farming the Earth had allowed the planet to harbour more and more people without humanity being struck by mass starvation.

But to Olsen, that explanation was too simple. He also believed himself to have observed Malthus's phenomenon with his own eyes. When, thanks to his all but extreme interest in rare birds, he'd first visited South Georgia — a small group of inaccessible islands between Argentina and Antarctica — the gentoo penguins had had 30,000 chicks. The following year, they'd had three. They simply ran out of food — in this case, krill.

It would be the same with humans. How many of us could the Earth really accommodate? The technical innovations stretching the planet's resources were only a temporary solution.

Björn Olsen eventually got his spot back in medical school, after an anatomy teacher put in a good word for him. And, as though by chance, it was this very combination of medical knowledge and an interest in animals that would see him go far.

Zoonoses

Despite all the years of medical research around the world, and all the billions of dollars poured into health campaigns, humanity has only ever managed to eradicate one single human infectious disease: smallpox.

The most important explanation is that smallpox is caused by a virus that only infects people: when there are no more infected humans left, the virus has nowhere to go.

But many of our best known diseases function differently. They are called zoonoses, or zoonotic diseases, and they spread between humans and animals. Transmission can happen directly — or via other animals. Such stopover animals are known as vectors. Often, these are ticks or insects. They suck blood from an infected animal, and might then go on to bite a person. That's how diseases such as tick-borne encephalitis (TBE) or malaria spread.

Influenza, rabies, HIV, Ebola, malaria, TBE, anthrax, salmonella — these are all zoonoses. Of the infectious diseases currently afflicting humanity, far beyond half originated in some animal.

It all starts with us humans disturbing an ecosystem, coming into contact with wild animals and disrupting their living environment. We do it because we want more resources, to consume things from the natural world: lumber, meat, minerals, and fossil fuels.

That's when viruses existing in apes, birds, or bats find a new host — us. It is no coincidence that the number of zoonotic disease outbreaks has increased at the same rate as the amount of untouched nature has dwindled.

Zoonoses: it sounds like a word out of a science fiction film. And that's pretty fitting, as zoonotic diseases belong to the future. A brutal future with more people and more diseases.

But Björn Olsen's misanthropy went even further. In his world, the phenomenon started as early as the domestication of animals during the Neolithic Revolution, when we managed to turn a small junglefowl from South-East Asia into the world's most common domestic bird, and when we raised more than a billion even-toed ungulates such as sheep, cows, and goats.

These monocultures may have been cost-effective, but they were also extremely sensitive to infectious diseases. A virus managing to break into chickens gained access to an almost boundless hunting ground; each chicken was like the next.

For every decade that passed after the Industrial Revolution, we made it easier and easier for new infections to spread. We built large-scale animal factories where viruses from wild birds could make a stopover, become more aggressive, and then jump back over to the wild birds again.

All that happened, Olsen thought, because there were so many of us. Because we needed more and more protein.

And the number of people was a danger in itself. We kept moving into increasingly crowded cities, travelled between them, and forced our way further and further into what had once been wilderness.

Björn Olsen was far from the only one to warn that our way of living would inevitably lead to further pandemics. In 2011, the film-maker Steven Soderbergh made *Contagion* — a film about a deadly virus spreading across the world. In the very last scene, the audience learns the origins of the disease: as an excavator mows down a forest, a bat is forced to flee towards a city and defecates on a domestic pig, which in turn gives the contagion to an Asian chef, who passes it on to Gwyneth Paltrow.

A year later, David Quammen's book was published, and the title — *Spillover* — described precisely what it was all about: diseases 'spilling over' from animals to humans.

Behind this budding cultural interest lay a worrying escalation of zoonotic diseases: the HIV epidemic in the 1980s, mad cow disease culminating in the 1990s, the 1997 avian flu, the 1999 Nipah virus, SARS in 2003, MERS in 2012.

But during these years the world had other problems, too: the Cold War, terrorism, climate change.

Biodiversity wasn't high up on the list.

Yet there was a group of people around the world interested in zoonoses. And its foremost Swedish representative was Björn Olsen.

His celebrity status in Sweden oscillated with the epidemics. If someone had had the idea of drawing up a graph plotting the times he'd been mentioned in the media, there would have been a strong correlation with the number of cases of influenza, SARS, or some other zoonosis.

It was the bird flu of 2006 that saw him raised to the nobility. Since the king of Sweden had long lost his right to confer nobility privileges, it was now Sweden's Radio that, each year, selected fifty or so particularly honourable Swedes to deliver an hour-long 'summer talk' on the radio.

The prize itself — telling semi-meaningless anecdotes from childhood for an hour, and perhaps selecting your own music — wasn't the thing. The thing was what it said about you as a person: you were a big deal.

And so this honour was bestowed on Björn Olsen back in 2006.

Three years later — in 2009 — the swine flu was spreading. It landed Olsen a book deal with the major Swedish publisher Norstedts. The book was given the title *Pandemic: myths, facts, threats*. It contained a prophecy about a new coronavirus: 'Imagine for a moment that SARS had behaved like a flu virus ten or a hundred times more infectious and with a fatality rate of a few per cent. That's a scenario we don't want to wake up to.'

When it came out the following year, however, public interest had waned.

The book fell into oblivion.

So it wasn't so strange that Björn Olsen was one of the first to pick up on what was happening in China at the start of 2020.

As early as 25 January, he'd warned in the daily newspaper *Svenska Dagbladet* that Sweden was unprepared for a large-scale virus outbreak. A week later, he advised Swedes not to travel to Asian countries.

Could this be the pandemic he'd been warning of for so long?

The schism

In Umeå, another expert on viruses was following the reports out of China. Fredrik Elgh wasn't as prone to worrying as Björn Olsen. More like the opposite.

Eleven years prior, in 2009, he had written an op-ed for the magazine *Journalisten* criticising one of Sweden's biggest daily newspapers, *Dagens Nyheter* — its science editor Karin Bojs, in particular — for unilaterally giving space to speculations and horror scenarios about a pandemic threat during both the avian flu and the swine flu, thus spreading unnecessary fear in society. Even though there was plenty of evidence to indicate that both epidemics were mild, *DN* and other media outlets had kept on beating the drum.

But this outbreak was different; the novel coronavirus simply couldn't be compared to a new flu. Against a flu, there were vaccines, antiviral drugs, and a certain resistance in people, built up as they'd come down with various influenzas throughout life. Possibly, it could be compared to the 'Asian flu' that raged in 1957 and the 'Hong Kong flu' that spread in Sweden in 1969. But back then, the healthcare system had been under a lot less strain. There had simply been more air in the system.

This could end badly. Fredrik Elgh did a quick multiplication off the top of his head: if half of all Swedes were infected, and 1 per cent of them died, that would result in 50,000 deaths.

In the last week of February, he began to compose a short op-ed. Even though there was still only one confirmed case in Sweden, he was certain the virus would soon be spreading far and wide in the country.

On 2 March, *Svenska Dagbladet* published his text. And now it was Fredrik Elgh's turn to use exclamation marks: 'As of yet no one can say exactly what this is going to look like. But one thing is certain. We must prepare for a worst-case scenario immediately!'

The same day, the Public Health Agency held a press conference in Stockholm. Director-General Johan Carlson outlined a 'worst possible scenario' in which 15,000 Swedes fell sick. The figures were based on an analysis of the number of hospitalisations in China. In Hubei Province (Wuhan is the capital city), between 1 and 1.5 people per thousand of the population had been affected. Translated into Swedish figures, that meant between 10,000 and 15,000 Swedes may find themselves in need of care.

Carlson also said there was much to indicate that Sweden would fare better than Hubei Province. Among the country's advantages was that it was more sparsely populated. That made it more likely that any outbreak would be smaller and limited to a geographical area.

At the same time, in Denmark, the Danish Health Authority assumed that more than half a million Danes might become infected. In Norway, the figures from the Norwegian Directorate of Health were even higher.

What looked like large differences between prognoses now began to be picked up by the media. *Dagens Nyheter*'s political commentator Ewa Stenberg called the state of information in Sweden 'confusing'.

'The Public Health Agency assumes a worst-case scenario where one out of every thousand in the population becomes infected. But Denmark bases its calculations on 10–15 per cent and Norway on 25 per cent of the population potentially becoming infected.'

The comparison was based on a misunderstanding, however — arising out of the way the Swedish Public Health Agency had chosen to calculate. While the Swedes were projecting the number of people 'falling sick' and thus requiring some form of care, Danish and Norwegian prognosticators were projecting the number of 'infections'.

Fredrik Elgh had known Anders Tegnell for a long time. Back in the day, Elgh had — at Johan Giesecke's suggestion — brought Anders Tegnell onto one of his teams and been his boss for a while. Among other things, they had been working together in 2001 when Sweden got its BSL-4 lab. The abbreviation was short for 'biosafety level 4', and it was the highest possible security classification for a laboratory. In such a lab, highly contagious pathogens were handled: Ebolaviruses, the variola virus, HFRS (hantavirus hemorrhagic fever with renal syndrome), and stuff like that. Only specially trained scientists were allowed access, and while conducting their work they had to wear pressure-regulated suits.

When Sweden first got its lab, there were only some thirty of them in the world; it was a source of national pride for the country's microbiologists and virologists.

Back then, Sweden was still a leading nation on infectious diseases. The government agency that during the course of the twentieth century changed its name from the National Medical Institution, via the National Bacteriological Laboratory, to the Swedish Institute for Infectious Disease Control had managed to suppress widespread diseases including tuberculosis, and to vaccinate away diphtheria, whooping cough, the measles, and mumps. It had churned out a polio vaccine that it shared with the entire world. It had played a central role in the eradication of smallpox.

It was a government agency like few others. It brought in money to the state treasury, and birthed some hundred doctoral theses — it even had a stable full of cows, horses, and monkeys so it could conduct its own animal testing.

'Few institutions in the world can pride themselves on having written a worthier chapter in the history of epidemiology,' an old head of the agency wrote in a memorial publication in honour of the National Bacteriological Laboratory published in 1993. Sweden, it was said, possessed a competence otherwise only found in the big international pharmaceutical industry.

There were differing views on how this legacy had been trifled away. Those who still remembered its heyday blamed meddlesome politicians — the kind that wanted to move government agencies into the outback. Others blamed jealous county councils or competing agencies; slowly, they'd stolen more and more of its tasks and resources.

From the year 2000, the Swedish Institute for Infectious Disease Control was governed by the doctor and microbiologist Ragnar Norrby — a person Fredrik Elgh liked, but who got caught up in a political brawl after eight years on the job. The background was the institute's refusal to help the police track down individuals infected with HIV. The minister for public health at the time, Maria Larsson, reprimanded Norrby and took the police's side. The next year, Norrby left his post, and in May 2009 Johan Carlson became the new director-general. Four years later,

Anders Tegnell was appointed as state epidemiologist at the agency. Now Swedish infectious-disease control was governed by two men who may have been doctors, but who'd long been working within the Swedish and European bureaucracies. Johan Carlson hadn't seen a patient since the beginning of the 1990s.

The recasting of the agency that Johan Giesecke had initiated by hiring more epidemiologists and statisticians now accelerated. Slowly, the microbiologists were pushed out.

Among those forced out was Jan Albert. He, too, was critical of the reorganisation. Albert thought it was a shame that the agency was divesting itself of its academic breadth, but at the same time he could understand the new leadership's thinking. Perhaps there had been a bit too much of a focus on basic research. Nor did he take it as personally as many others.

Fredrik Elgh watched these developments with dismay. For a while, he and a few other microbiologists considered setting up their own reference lab.

Eventually, the existing expertise was divvied up between a few different universities: sexually transmitted diseases ended up in Örebro, hepatitis research in Gothenburg, and HFRS in Umeå.

It actually worked out pretty well, Elgh thought much later. But his schism with the new regime at the Institute for Infectious Disease Control continued with unabated force. One of the discussions concerned the human papillomavirus, or HPV. It was a virus that caused cervical cancer, but also anal cancer, cancer in the pharyngeal region, and cancer in the sex organs.

In the fall of 2013, Sweden began to vaccinate all girls in Year Five against the virus — but not the boys of the same age. Fredrik Elgh thought that was stupid.

The mistrust between the country's leadership on infectious-disease control and a large number of its microbiologists seemed to grow with each passing year.

This antagonism didn't exist only in Sweden. In several infectious-disease control agencies around the world, there was a conflict between those who peered deep into their microscopes and those who preferred to look at the bigger picture.

On 1 January 2014, Sweden chose a strategy in that battle. That day, the Swedish Institute for Infectious Disease Control was closed down and absorbed by a new agency: the Public Health Agency of Sweden.

Behind this reorganisation lay modern ideas about a holistic approach to public health. The fight against viruses and bacteria was now part of a much wider effort to create a healthier population. At the same time, the work on infectious-disease control was condensed into a single location. Tasks previously falling to the National Board of Health and Welfare were now moved to the new agency.

The government agency born on that day was largely Johan Carlson's creation. He was the one who had led the special investigation that preceded the reformation, and now he became its first director-general.

After Fredrik Elgh's op-ed on 2 March, the microbiologist diaspora began to rally. They created a long email thread, which kept on growing and growing. In it, they criticised the lack of competence at the Public Health Agency.

Many on the email thread specialised in molecular research, but pretty soon the group had widened to include mathematicians and other epidemiologists.

One of the epidemiologists was Joacim Rocklöv, an academic wonderchild and budding talent at Umeå University. He mainly researched the impact of climate change on health.

But the biggest name without a doubt was Björn Olsen. With every alarming report coming out of China, his pandemic book was now selling more and more copies. His publisher had to order additional print runs. He was constantly on TV.

Once again, his celebrity status tracked the curve of an infectious disease.

Olsen and Elgh had known each other for a long time. They had gone to medical school one term apart and had followed each other's work throughout the years; after all, they both specialised in infectious diseases. Olsen had a summer cottage outside Umeå, where Elgh lived. So sometimes they'd see each other in the summer.

Moreover, Björn Olsen had had his own scuffles with the Institute for Infectious Disease Control and the Public Health Agency. His book was full of little jibes about, as well as more explicit attacks on, those conceited Stockholmers. He thought they'd been slow to work out a pandemic strategy, and was critical of their stance against building a national vaccine factory. Living in Stockholm was almost a risk factor, in Olsen's mind. Like many others, he was deeply interested in the Spanish flu — and even then, 102 years ago, the Stockholm bureaucracy had been slow to act at the start of the pandemic.

So far, no one knew with certainty how hard the new virus would hit Sweden. The WHO had not yet declared the world overtaken by a new pandemic. Any deaths connected to the new virus had not yet been registered in Sweden.

But now there was at least an opposition — all ready and set — against the people at the helm of the Public Health Agency.

Björn Olsen, Fredrik Elgh, and the other scientists planned to act. In their emails, they were discussing a 'battle plan'.

They'd waited a long time.

Now they were striking back.

A dry-land swimmer

When Tom Britton returned from France, he took up Julia Gog's exhortation: he got to work full-time on the new virus.

This was new to him. Most diseases he'd worked on in the past had really only consisted of interchangeable Greek letters. When he'd made calculations about a certain disease, its characteristics had been distilled into their mathematical constituent parts: incubation time, rate of transmission, level of immunity. About symptoms and the stuff doctors dealt with — what happened in the real world to those who got sick — he knew very little. He learnt, but forgot.

It was as though he wasn't very interested.

Two diseases he knew a bit more about: AIDS and hepatitis C. On those, he had contributed with a few conclusions in the form of numbers. But to a Swede, it was almost like studying history. Cases of hepatitis C had been falling since the beginning of the 1990s, and HIV was big in the 1980s.

The new virus was spreading *now* — as he was writing his code and calculations. There were more and more cases all the time.

Was it going to reach Sweden?

He had never been in a rush like this before.

He felt like he had been practising dry-land swimming for 25 years. Now he was in the water.

Unlike Anders Tegnell and Lisa Brouwers, Tom Britton thought it was possible to use MacDonald's reproduction number to calculate the spread of infection. The fact that the virus was spreading globally through clusters was of no significance for the models. If 90 people didn't transmit the virus to anyone, and 10 people each passed it on to 15 others, that didn't mean there were two different values for R_0. Instead, you added up the total transmission. If so, those 100 had transmitted the virus to a total of 150 people — giving it an R_0 of 1.5.

The figures indicating the proportion of people who had got sick in Wuhan didn't really say much about how the virus would behave in

Europe. After all, the Chinese had engaged the entire arsenal of their dictatorship to clamp down on the virus.

According to Britton's calculations, R_0 for the coronavirus was between 2 and 2.5. He had arrived at this number by observing how quickly the death toll rose and then combining that figure with estimates of the virus's generation time, which had begun to be published here and there.

Between 2 and 2.5 — this meant the virus was very likely to sweep over Sweden.

Around this time, reports also began to come in about how hard northern Italy was being hit. The way Britton saw it, the fact that it was Italy, of all places, was an accident of fate; they just happened to get the virus first in Europe. Now he felt that radical changes were needed to the way Swedish people behaved.

In the first week of March, the situation was becoming acute. The February break was over, and between 2 and 6 March thousands of children in Stockholm — just returned from Italy, Austria, and France — would go back to school as usual.

It wasn't just doctors and epidemiologists who were sounding the alarm. The political editor-in-chief at *Dagens Nyheter*, Amanda Sokolnicki, wrote on Twitter that these children being told to go back to school as usual was 'incomprehensible'.

The measures introduced by the Public Health Agency around this time were of an almost surgical nature: only people feeling sick and who had also been to China, South Korea, Hong Kong, Iran, or northern Italy should contact the healthcare services. Only flights from Iran had been suspended.

Tom Britton wanted to see broader interventions. Because the testing capacity was so low in many countries, no one could really be certain of how many had been infected.

He thought the agency should advise all Swedes to take their bikes instead of riding the Metro to work, avoid hugging for a while, and wash their hands more regularly. The most important thing was to get onto the media right away and tell everyone with any kind of symptoms to stay home, with immediate effect.

Moreover, these measures were more or less without cost, and very easy to implement. Especially in comparison with the costs that could arise if the worst-case scenarios from his calculations came true.

From China, reports were emerging about the regime imposing a curfew in several parts of the country. Hundreds of thousands of volunteers and representatives from the Communist Party were helping to isolate cities and taking citizens' temperatures. The country's leader, Xi Jinping, called it a 'people's war' against the virus, and it reminded many Chinese of the Red Guards who had gone around terrorising their countrymen during the Cultural Revolution.

In the foreign media, the Chinese strategy began to be referred to as a 'lockdown' — a complete shutdown of society.

Considering that the deadliness did not appear particularly extreme, Britton thought China's strategy seemed needlessly harsh. But, at the same time, he thought the Swedish Public Health Agency was taking the threat a little too lightly. By 2 March, the agency had updated its assessment once more, but the risk of community transmission was still deemed moderate.

Tom Britton knew he wasn't the only one in Sweden who saw what was about to happen. He'd read Fredrik Elgh's article. He'd heard what Björn Olsen had to say. He'd read the papers. But he wasn't like the other whistleblowers. Of all the outsiders with opinions about the agency's actions, Britton had a unique position.

Most of all, he had a contact in Johan Giesecke. Tom's father — the infectious-disease specialist Sven Britton — had known Giesecke for decades. Together with Johan, Tom Britton had founded the Stockholm Group for Epidemic Modeling, to which, for instance, Lisa Brouwers was connected.

Of the four people working at the agency's unit for analysis, moreover, one had been Britton's doctoral supervisee, and he'd published scientific articles with another. He still saw them every now and then through their 'journal club'. It was like a book club where they met to discuss scientific articles on mathematics and statistics. In addition, Britton was in close contact with some of the doctors and experts in the agency's immediate orbit.

With Anders Tegnell, things were a bit more complicated. They had indeed met several times at different conferences; but, as Britton recalled, Tegnell had always left the meetings early because of some urgent phone call. So he was a bit unsure whether he really knew the state epidemiologist.

On the morning of 6 March, Tom Britton sent his first email to Anders Tegnell. He could sense it wouldn't pay to criticise him too much. He knew those who did hadn't got anywhere.

He struck a humble tone.

'Busy days for you. Here are some thoughts from someone who isn't quite as up to speed on reality, but who is on infectious-disease modelling.'

He made no secret of his belief that the Public Health Agency was being too passive: 'With as many cases as there now are in Sweden, the disease will spread. Our society isn't all that different from Italy, or China for that matter, so why wouldn't it spread here?'

There was a lot Britton didn't write. He knew there were only four people in the unit for analysis, and it bugged him that the agency hadn't had the foresight to bring more experts into its network. In a crisis like this, it would have allowed them to mobilise an entire crew of statisticians and analysts.

Instead, he ended on a note of half praise, half warning: 'I think you have been wise not to paint the devil on the wall, but nevertheless we all have to be prepared that with an $R_0>2$, 80 per cent will be infected unless we do something.'

Britton also knew what he didn't know. This was a world of unknown figures multiplied by more unknown figures. Though he feared a large-scale outbreak in Sweden, he was also aware that the outcome could end up being less severe. If one of the variables was bigger or smaller than he'd assumed, it could have substantial consequences for the end results.

What should be done with the information the mathematical models spat back out wasn't clear. It depended on how much risk you were willing to accept, what type of person you were.

Tom Britton didn't know it yet, but in that respect he and Anders Tegnell were different — very different.

The mathematician now hitting the 'send' button was a person who always wore a helmet when riding his bike.

The state epidemiologist receiving the email biked without a helmet.

Britton waited tensely in front of the computer. Three hours later, Tegnell replied: 'Happy to discuss this further.'

Tom Britton was in.

Three doctors

And so, late on Friday 6 March, Jan Albert, Johan von Schreeb, and Denis Coulombier sat facing Anders Tegnell in an empty dining hall.

The table they were seated around was illuminated by a cone-shaped lamp. With its uncomfortable wooden chairs, slight industrial feel, and depressing view over winter-bare trees and a parking lot, it could have been any canteen in any government agency anywhere in Sweden.

The first week of March was coming to an end. Anders Tegnell's stoic attitude towards the new virus had been attacked from all directions imaginable.

It wasn't just the usual band of microbiologists — Björn Olsen, Fredrik Elgh, and others always critical of the agency. It was Tom Britton. It was *Dagens Nyheter*'s editorial page. It was scientists at the universities in Umeå and Uppsala. It was doctors all over the country questioning his thinking when he advised medical personnel who'd been to Italy over the break to go back to work.

'The Public Health Agency and the healthcare services [believe] that symptoms of Covid-19 as though by some miracle always make their first appearance outside of working hours,' chief physician Anders Jansson wrote in an op-ed for the medical trade publication *Läkartidningen*.

In the comments below the text, doctors across the country aired their discontent with both Tegnell and the agency. And this wasn't like the trolls on social media. These doctors signed with their names, titles, workplaces — everything.

They were pissed off, quite simply. And they weren't ashamed to show it.

In the rest of the world, the restrictions grew more and more numerous. Italy and Japan had closed their schools. In France, students who returned from vacations abroad were encouraged to stay home for two weeks. In Germany, all who crossed the country's border by plane or train were being registered.

Around the world, discussions now began about even tougher interventions: closed borders, travel restrictions, full-on curfews.

But in the deserted dining hall outside Sweden's capital, Anders Tegnell resisted.

Denis Coulombier looked at the state epidemiologist. He'd been sure that his, von Schreeb's, and Albert's advice about imposing restrictions would be heeded. After all, what they'd presented was so overwhelming.

The state epidemiologist continued to speak. He wasn't just unwilling to close schools. He also seemed to think it unnecessary to tell Swedes to change their behaviour in any major way.

Imposing restrictions during an epidemic was a matter of timing. If you did it too soon — when there were only a few cases — the epidemic would simply start all over again once the restrictions were lifted.

These differing views on the new virus — represented this Friday in the agency's dining hall by Coulombier and Tegnell — existed all over the world. In the rooms where decisions were now being made — in the US, the UK, and Sweden — two diverging viewpoints were pitted against each other: go with your gut, or trust the data?

Should they be putting their faith in abstract mathematical models, snapshots from the chaos in Italy, and shaky mortality figures from China? Or in the numbers showing that the spread of the virus in Sweden remained low?

Many of the measures already implemented or planned in other countries were incredibly costly — both for economic and social reasons. Anders Tegnell wasn't the kind of man who made that type of decision based on a vague 'gut feeling', no matter how many doctors and professors came knocking and tried to persuade him otherwise.

This was the tenacity that Giesecke had once fallen for.

Part II

Of mice and sticks

In the early twentieth century, the study of epidemics had become more and more of an indoors job.

It wasn't all that strange. The bacteriological revolution had given humanity both vaccines and insight into the value of washing your hands. So what was the point of looking elsewhere?

In order to understand diseases, you needed a lab — or at least a microscope.

The future was in the microscope. And yet it didn't let you see everything. Because in spite of all this new knowledge about viruses, bacteria, and parasites, there were lots of phenomena that couldn't be explained about the diseases plaguing mankind.

Why didn't everyone fall sick in a severe epidemic? Why did the outbreaks appear to follow a characteristic curve?

For a long time, many doctors and epidemiologists had explained the eventual decline of any epidemic with a theory that the virus or bacteria was weakened with every person it passed through. As though each person was a little filter. The disease entered on one side and came out on the other, a little weaker. But thanks to Ronald Ross and his mosquito theorem, there was no need for an assumption about pathogens gradually growing weaker. Instead, there appeared to be a threshold. When the number of infected individuals rose above it, the epidemic died out.

There seemed to be a complexity in the way infections spread. Something social. Something almost magical.

Somewhere in there was a mathematical law.

In New York in the 1920s, the scientist Leslie T. Webster designed a series of ingenious experiments to find out what was really happening when a disease spread through a population. In a room at the Rockefeller Institute, he built a tiny city of mice. He put out cages — with five healthy mice in each — and fed them the same food every day: grains in the morning, and bread dunked in milk in the afternoon.

He was also careful to keep the room clean of any bugs or vermin. The cages were thoroughly cleaned once a week and the temperature kept at a consistent 20 degrees Celsius.

It was, in other words, a fairly pleasant existence for the mice — until Webster began to infect them with typhoid.

Carefully and methodically, Webster and his colleagues infected them with the bacterium causing typhoid in mice. Sometimes one at a time; sometimes more. Maintaining a true scientific spirit, Webster changed one small circumstance at a time, while keeping all other factors consistent.

And perhaps this was a bit unlucky. His thoroughness — which in other cases would have been an asset — made the experiment somewhat meaningless.

After all, that's not how diseases spread. There is no divine hand giving out diseases to one mouse at a time, like Webster's laboratory assistants.

Nor was the environment he'd built particularly natural. In the book *Heredity and Infection: the history of disease transmission*, historian of science Olga Amsterdamska writes that the living environment of the New York mice was closer to a prison, or at best a boring American suburb.

Around the same time in London, another mouse community was being built. Its architect was named William Whiteman Carlton Topley.

Topley was a bacteriologist at the London School of Tropical Hygiene, and, like Webster in New York, he harboured suspicions about the magical way that diseases spread and suddenly went away again.

Topley, too, worked on mice — only a slightly more urban kind. Instead of isolating them in smaller cages, he let the mice run around in one single, giant cage. In other words, they lived more like people in Europe at the time: in densely populated communities. Topley thought his mouse community resembled a monastery; sometimes there were novices, and the only way out was to die.

Perhaps that wasn't entirely accurate. After all, mice behave quite differently from monks and nuns: they eat each other, mate, and kill their own offspring.

So just as soon as Topley had come up with the analogy of the monastery, he rejected it. This was, he admitted, an artificial environment.

And yet it led him to several insights. When Topley infected the mice with potentially deadly bacteria, he noticed that the composition of the mouse population determined how many died.

If all the mice were healthy and none were immune, they all died within a few weeks. But when Topley mixed in a few immunised mice, quite a few of them survived — even among the mice that hadn't been immune from the start.

'The question of immunity as an attribute of a herd should be studied as a separate problem,' he wrote in a 1923 article titled 'The Spread of Bacterial Infection. The Problem of Herd Immunity'.

Herd immunity. This was the first time the term had been mentioned in the scientific literature. But how herd immunity worked was less clear. What kind of phenomenon was this?

A few years later, in 1926, Topley attempted yet another analogy. Imagine a bunch of sticks: some of them are thick, others thin. We push all of them into the ground. Then we begin to throw rocks at them. The rocks are all different, too. Some are heavy; others are light. And each throw is unique. Sometimes we throw hard; other times less so. Sometimes we hit our target; sometimes we miss.

That's how an infection spreads, Topley thought. It's not just mice and people that are unique. Like the rocks being thrown, each incident of transmission has varying mass and velocity.

After a while, we'll have knocked some of the sticks over. The thickest still stand, but also some of the thinnest. Around them, Topley wrote, protective piles of 'ineffective missiles' have formed.

It was a brilliant analogy. Or it would have been — had it been true.

Topley came far with his urban mice. But he didn't come all the way.

There was something about social interactions that caused epidemics to taper off, disappear, and then return again.

But what was happening?

A few years after Topley's experiments with mice, a doctor under the name of A.W. Hedrich started keeping a balance sheet of the number of measles cases and newborns in the city of Baltimore on the American east coast.

Like many other parts of the world, Baltimore was hit by fairly regular epidemics. Around every other or every third year, measles swept through the city. At first glance, there didn't appear to be any consistency in the number of cases. Sometimes there were many; sometimes few.

But through his calculations, Hedrich could determine what proportion of children was susceptible to the disease at any moment in time. And suddenly he noticed a pattern: just before the outbreak of any large measles epidemic, the proportion of susceptible children under the age of 15 was between 45 and 50 per cent. Once the epidemic was over, the same figure had dropped to between 30 and 35 per cent.

The relationship between the number of immune and susceptible children thus moved within a narrow range.

It seemed as though measles epidemics couldn't take off if enough children were immune. It brought to mind Ronald Ross — the doctor in love with mathematics — and his mosquito theorem. But this involved no reservoirs of mosquitoes; the disease spread directly from one person to another.

What was actually happening?

Topley's analogy about the sticks and the rocks had almost hit the mark. But it wasn't the ineffective rocks that allowed the weak sticks to stay standing. It was the strong sticks that were the protection. With enough of them, the rocks couldn't reach the weak sticks. It was as though the susceptible individuals — mice, sticks, children — were protected by an almost impenetrable wall.

Hedrich concluded that there was a cut-off point at 55 per cent. If that many children were immune against the disease, it couldn't gain any momentum.

There lay the threshold for herd immunity.

Now forget that number. Immediately. Wipe it from your memory. Achieving herd immunity against measles requires levels of more than 90 per cent.

But whatever. This was almost a century ago, and we mustn't let a minor — okay, rather major — miscalculation diminish Hedrich's big insight.

Think of the number as *Kitty Hawk*, the airplane the Wright brothers successfully launched into the air in 1903 and whose flight can be watched in grainy black-and-white YouTube videos.

That's not an aeroplane you want a seat on. But who cares? It flew.

You see, the thing about Hedrich's percentage wasn't the number itself — but the very idea that such a figure existed.

The notion that for every infectious disease there is a herd-immunity level — which can be calculated in advance — would have big consequences.

100 per cent mortality

Two things were mainly said about Johan Giesecke: that he was exceptionally smart and exceptionally self-confident. These two attributes no one disputed. Instead, it was the balance between them, the direction in which the scales tipped, that determined the view people took of him.

There were those who thought he was a brilliant, polyglot Renaissance man. And there were those who described him as a bit too brash, a bit too cocksure.

Over the years, his self-assurance had developed from a character trait into a professional strategy. He'd noticed there was an advantage in conveying confidence and authority.

One thing was certain: Johan Giesecke was a man with many thoughts and opinions. Both big and small.

Among the small ones was his desire to eradicate the semi-colon from the Swedish language. 'All they do is show you've been to college,' he'd say, quoting the writer Kurt Vonnegut.

He'd jotted down one of his more serious ideas and sent it to the national daily newspaper *Dagens Nyheter* in April 1992. The text had the title 'Don't Listen to the Medical Sciences!' — exclamation mark and all. In it, he explained that society and its citizens had misunderstood the reasons why we live so much longer these days. It wasn't primarily because of medical conquests, such as new drugs or new ways of operating on people — it was thanks to clean water, sewerage systems, sufficient food, better housing.

Society is the reason we live as long as we do: democracy, a market economy, institutions. Which countries had the fewest cases of cervical cancer among women in the EU? The rich ones.

There was something unsound about the way doctors within certain disciplines proclaimed that their disease above others killed the most people. That was no way to think, argued Giesecke, who was by this time an associate professor in infectious diseases. For if, somehow, we magically eradicated high cholesterol levels, this would indeed lower the mortality of cardiovascular disease. But it would only make the 'risk' of dying of cancer go up.

It was a text made for printing out in a large font, framing, and hanging among the wine bottles in a bar: 'You should be careful about changing a way of life that you enjoy, or starting a lifelong preventative treatment, simply because research finds that it could help with a specific disease.'

When Johan Giesecke gave lectures, he would say the mortality rate in Sweden was 100 per cent. It wasn't so much an opinion as a fact, but it lent some insight into his thinking on life and death. As he wrote in that article: 'If we can prevent people from dying of this disease, what will it be that kills them instead?'

'History books are watching us'

On the afternoon of 8 March, Tom Britton emailed Anders Tegnell with yet another set of arguments as to why Sweden should introduce several new recommendations immediately.

Because Britton assumed the virus had already established itself in the country, it was now a matter of how the uninfected should behave: he wanted the agency to call on Swedes not to take the bus or the Metro, to avoid crowds, and not to shake hands or hug.

'One relevant question,' he wrote, 'is whether it's worth making an effort to lower R if you don't expect to be able to push it below 1.'

Was it worth getting the R number down — perhaps from 3 to 2 — Britton asked rhetorically.

'Looking at the end results, the number of infections drops from something like 85 per cent to 70 per cent. Is it worth the effort?'

The way he saw it, the unequivocal answer was yes. He attached two graphs to illustrate the difference.

'Firstly, the height of the peak is much lower, which is important when thinking about the strain on hospitals. And the peak also comes with a delay, which means more time to prepare.'

But Tegnell wasn't sold. He wrote back: 'If we're looking at flu pandemics, that type of effort has had an extremely limited impact of possibly a few days' delay and perhaps a somewhat flattened peak. Experiences from China might possibly indicate that corona is more malleable, and the way things develop in Italy may tell us something about that.'

They emailed back and forth. Anders Tegnell argued there was little evidence to indicate that the recommendations would really help.

Britton turned sour.

'So all that is left to do then is wait until we find ourselves in Italy's position and proceed to lock down Stockholm, Gothenburg, etc? Sounds to my ears like a much too pessimistic attitude, and psychologically inappropriate too.'

Ten minutes later, Tegnell replied: 'No, that wouldn't work communicatively of course.'

Jan Albert was also upping the pressure. He bombarded Tegnell with various studies showing a need for stronger measures. But despite sending his objections to those in charge at the agency, Albert chose to keep his comments within a limited sphere. By now, the coronavirus was dominating the news in Sweden, and, as a professor of infectious-disease control, Jan Albert was invited to go on television almost daily.

The criticism against Anders Tegnell had become increasingly loud. But Albert decided not to join in the chorus. The way he saw it, Sweden was now facing a huge challenge, and in such a situation it was important to restore confidence in the Public Health Agency.

He started emailing Anders Tegnell ahead of his own TV appearances, telling him what he'd say.

Yet the trend was clear. Slowly but surely, Tom Britton and Jan Albert began to wear down the resistance inside the Public Health Agency.

On 11 March, the government — based on a recommendation from the agency — issued a ban on gatherings of more than 500 people. At the same time, recommendations were being drafted on working from home in Stockholm, as well as on remote teaching for upper-secondary schools and universities.

The debate about whether Sweden would be hit was over. Jan Albert felt pleased, and thought the matter resolved.

Tom Britton, too, thought the Public Health Agency was on the right track. Because the virus wasn't extremely deadly, it was hard to justify tough restrictions on people's lives. He didn't believe in closing schools at all.

Slowly, a new unanimity began to form between the state epidemiologist, the mathematician, and the professor of infectious-disease control.

At the same time, the three doctors who had walked together to the Public Health Agency to warn Anders Tegnell less than a week previously were beginning to drift apart. Gradually, they began to form different opinions about what measures were required to face the looming pandemic.

The next day, 12 March, Denis Coulombier wrote in an email to Jan Albert and Johan von Schreeb that he hoped 'Anders & Co.' would act swiftly. It was time to close the schools.

'History books are watching us,' the Frenchman wrote.

But from now on, the Swedes in the group would fall in with Tegnell's line — which was also theirs. In short, its main gist was that it was reasonable to make certain simple interventions, but closing down schools — or society, for that matter — would be an overreaction.

What no one foresaw was that the rest of the world was about to side with the Frenchman.

'Don't you know, my son, with how little wisdom the world is governed?'

Johan Giesecke's return to the Public Health Agency happened gradually in early March 2020. It started with Anders Tegnell asking if he'd like to be part of an expert group on the new virus. Giesecke said yes, and immediately got to work relaying his knowledge and opinions to his protégé.

On 11 March, Giesecke received some figures from an Italian epidemiologist called Alessandro Cassini. Cassini had once worked under Giesecke at the ECDC, but now he was back in Italy.

Among other things, the figures sent by the Italian indicated that many of those who'd been infected in Italy didn't show any symptoms whatsoever.

Giesecke forwarded the information to Tegnell.

This was interesting.

The fact that there were infected individuals who didn't display symptoms was by now fairly well known among doctors and epidemiologists. But what implications these asymptomatic people had for the spread of the disease wasn't clear. One week prior, the ECDC had arrived at the conclusion that those who didn't display any symptoms also couldn't pass it on to someone else. But no one knew for certain. It was clear, however, that a majority of those who got it displayed only mild symptoms — 80 per cent, according to the calculations they had received from the ECDC.

Here, Johan Giesecke's and Anders Tegnell's estimates began to diverge. Giesecke thought there were already thousands of infections in Sweden; Tegnell believed the number to be a lot lower.

Despite this, Giesecke wasn't particularly worried. Quite the opposite. If the rate of transmission was so high, with so many not showing symptoms, Sweden had already entered the so-called pandemic phase, involving widespread infection and a large number of cases. It meant there was no point engaging in contact tracing.

In other words, the virus was like a storm sweeping across the country. It wouldn't subside until enough people had been infected and become immune. It would take a month or two, and then Sweden would have achieved herd immunity against the virus.

The ban on gatherings of more than 500 people was a measure requested by the Public Health Agency — but Giesecke didn't like the idea. If they thought it was an effective restriction, the limit had to be set much lower. Perhaps as low as ten people.

Just as pointless was the ban on travel to Sweden introduced by the government. Every country already had its own community transmission. The storm was already here. What remained to be done now was to protect the most vulnerable groups in society.

'It's becoming time to think about how to introduce bans on visits to nursing homes,' Johan Giesecke wrote to Anders Tegnell.

'It's on the list,' Tegnell replied.

During this time, there was also a discussion about whether to keep schools open for children in Years One to Nine. Closing schools was an intervention that had been used since the time of the Spanish flu. As recently as during the 2009 swine flu, more than 700 schools had closed for a time in the US.

There were multiple reasons many thought it was a good idea. During flu epidemics, children tended to be the ones driving the spread of infection. Besides, it was an efficient way of making social life freeze overnight. When children stayed home, at least one parent had to as well.

A study published in the journal *Nature* in 2006 had showed that closing schools at the right time could flatten the curve and limit the strain on the healthcare system.

In 2009, the British journal *The Lancet* had published an article with the title 'Closure of Schools During an Influenza Pandemic'. It covered several historical scenarios: the Spanish flu of 1918, the 1957 Asian flu, a 2008 outbreak of bird flu in Hong Kong, and a few other pandemics. One of its seven authors was Anders Tegnell. But no clear recommendations were to be found, even for a close reader. On the one hand, there was some historical support for closing schools. Experiences in France and the US showed that the number of cases could 'maybe' be reduced by 15 per cent in an optimistic scenario. At the same time, those gains were likely to be lost if the children weren't completely isolated when staying home from school.

And the intervention came at a high cost. The bill for closing British schools for 12 weeks was estimated at 1 per cent of the country's GDP in the *Lancet* article. In the US, an equivalent intervention would cost 6 per cent of GDP. And as school closures would also force many doctors and nurses to stay home from their jobs, that consequence had to be weighed up, too.

It was a hard nut to crack. But not for Johan Giesecke. He was completely convinced it was the wrong route to take.

Most of all, he thought, it would be unfair on the children. He recalled studies he'd read about school absences having an adverse effect on children's living conditions well into later life.

Besides, the pandemic that the world was now living through seemed different from an influenza epidemic. As yet there was little data, but judging by experiences from China, children weren't the ones driving the transmission. So far, they hadn't seen a single outbreak in a school.

In Sweden, as in many other countries, a large majority of healthcare workers were women. If the schools were barred up, many women would stay home with their children. Say there was, on average, two kids per family, he reasoned. If so, would half a million people have to stay home from work?

There were plenty of anecdotes from epidemiological history to lean on. During the Spanish flu, the legendary New York City Board of Health president, Royal S. Copeland, had kept schools open throughout the pandemic.

Copeland had received harsh criticism, but defended his decision by arguing that the alternative was even more dangerous from an infectious-disease standpoint: 'If the schools were closed, at least 1,000,000 would be sent to their homes and become 1,000,000 possibilities for the disease. Furthermore, there would be nobody to take special notice of their condition.'

Schools were part of society, of the system that the world's countries had built up over centuries to maintain public health. That was the view Copeland had held. And that was the view held by Johan Giesecke 102 years later.

Giesecke spent his mornings in phone meetings with a group of experts put together by Jan Albert. Among these scientists and doctors, many wanted to close the schools. In uncharacteristic fashion, Giesecke mostly sat there listening during those meetings. They weren't the people he needed to convince. The one holding the power was Anders Tegnell.

On Wednesday 11 March came the first setback. At a late press conference in Copenhagen, the Danish prime minister, Mette Fredriksen, declared that all preschools, schools, and universities in Denmark would close the following Monday.

At 2.00 pm the next day, Thursday 12 March, Norway followed suit.

Prime Minister Erna Solberg announced that all schools in the country would close, as would all hair salons, tattoo studios, and similar businesses. All organised sports would cease, too. These interventions were described as the most pervasive ever to be implemented in Norway during peacetime.

The Norwegian infection control director, Frode Forland, had once worked under Johan Giesecke at the ECDC. They knew each other well. But it was the Norwegian politicians, not the Norwegian Institute of Public Health, who had made the decision.

Now the pressure on Sweden mounted. That same afternoon, the minister for education, Anna Ekström, sat down for a meeting with representatives of school principals and government agencies. A press conference had been promised for eight o'clock that evening.

Among the journalists who waited, most expected Sweden to follow its Nordic neighbours.

When Anna Ekström finally emerged and delivered her verdict, she explained that there were no legal obstacles to closing schools in Sweden, but that the government had chosen not to: 'It's a clear recommendation from the Public Health Agency, and they are very keen to see it followed.'

One journalist wanted to know why Sweden wasn't doing the same as Denmark and Norway.

Ekström replied like Giesecke would have: 'My strongest argument is that if mums and dads working in the healthcare systems have to stay home with their children, the healthcare services will suffer.'

Johan Giesecke had won the first battle. But holding his ground would be hard. It was clear that the governments of the world had been struck by panic. Early the next morning, Giesecke sent an email to Anders Tegnell. He wrote, in italics: '*An nescis, mi fili, quantilla prudentia mundus regatur.*'

These were words that the Swedish high chancellor Axel Oxenstierna was said to have once written in a letter to his son, Johan Oxenstierna. As the myth goes, his son was feeling nervous ahead of a trip to the peace talks in Westphalia in the 1640s.

Now it was Giesecke who sent the words to his own boy, as he, too, had been drawn into international politics.

Just to be safe, he added a translation: 'Don't you know, my son, with how little wisdom the world is governed?'

Where the bureaucrats rule

About a year before the novel coronavirus began its journey from China out into the rest of the world, the Swedish minister for home affairs, Mikael Damberg, journeyed a few blocks through Stockholm — from the Swedish Government Offices to the large building on Kungsholmen where Sweden's leading police officers worked.

It was 21 February 2019. The minister had brought with him a list of things he wanted the police to prioritise. It included cracking down on gross violence, increasing the number of officers on duty, and other things.

In other words, these were no controversial tasks he wanted the police to carry out. By this time, a synthesis of migration, social exclusion, and serious crime had become the biggest — perhaps only — political issue in Sweden, so the items on the list were not particularly surprising.

But a month later, the legal policy spokesman for the Moderate Party, Johan Forssell, found out about the meeting. This was not acceptable, he told the media. A minister mustn't micromanage a government agency this way.

He was now considering reporting Mikael Damberg to the parliamentary committee on the constitution. This might be a matter of 'ministerial rule'.

Accusations of 'ministerial rule' are a never-ending saga in Swedish politics. It's probably one of the most misused terms in the whole of the Swedish language. It has served both as a weapon and an excuse, and few seem able to define what it means.

Yet it speaks to a unique detail in the Swedish constitution. Take, for instance, the minister for home affairs and his police force. In all the world's countries, it's pretty much a given that the minister responsible for the police is allowed to tell it what to do.

But not in Sweden.

There are autonomous body parts in all forms of government. In democracies, the courts are typically independent. For several decades, moats have been dug between central banks and elected politicians. And in certain types of democracies, power is divided between a legislative and an executive branch.

What's unique about Sweden is that government agencies are independent, too. So if the government wants, say, the Swedish Migration Agency to do something, they can't call up the director-general and give him an order. In some cases, this would even be illegal. Under the Swedish constitution, neither the government nor the parliament may 'determine how an administrative authority shall decide in a particular case relating to the exercise of public authority vis-à-vis an individual or a local authority, or relating to the application of law'.

The Swedish government has indirect ways of making agencies do its will: changing their appropriation directions, or appointing heads of agencies. It also has the power to close down or merge agencies.

It's a system more reminiscent of the way the board of a company might draw up an overall strategy and appoint a CEO — but then lets the CEO run the company in whatever way that person sees fit.

Sitting in a room without windows on Herkulesgatan in Stockholm was the GSS — the Group for Strategic Coordination. These were the people who led the government's handling of the pandemic.

That it was the specific people in this room who ended up in charge of handling the pandemic was a bit of an accident.

It was the result of several different circumstances.

Since the 2014 elections, Stefan Löfven had been Sweden's prime minister. Unlike many of his predecessors, Löfven hadn't actively sought the job as the leader of the Social Democratic Party — and thereby its candidate for prime minister. After the party had gone through both internal strife and two failed party leaders in succession, he had been persuaded to run as a compromise candidate.

As prime minister, Löfven was fairly withdrawn. He wasn't the kind of person who sought the limelight for no reason. In one of his first decisions as prime minister, he passed crisis management from his own office over to the Ministry of Justice. This was in part due to Löfven's penchant for delegating. But also to the fact that, in the same move, he set up a position as minister for home affairs under the Ministry of Justice. That job went to Anders Ygeman, who was thereby promoted as perhaps the biggest future name within the Social Democratic Party.

But in the summer of 2017, Ygeman was forced to resign after it became known that the Swedish Transport Agency had allowed personnel abroad without security clearances to process sensitive information from the Swedish driving licence register, among others places. Instead, Mikael Damberg became minister for home affairs. And so it was his state secretary who, in the winter of 2020, was tasked with leading GSS and handling the pandemic. Her name was Elisabeth Backteman, she was 53 years old, and she was a bit of an anonymous figure in the political world.

But the group also included a few other — significantly more powerful — individuals: the state secretary to the prime minister, Nils Vikmång; the head of press, Odd Guteland; the state secretary for foreign affairs, Robert Rydberg; and the state secretary to the minister for finance, Emma Lennartsson.

Of this, however, few Swedes were aware.

It wasn't all that strange. After all, it was Anders Tegnell or some other official who, like a true father or mother of the nation, would drone on at the daily press conference at 2.00 pm from some room in Solna.

Not Prime Minister Stefan Löfven. Nor anyone else in the government.

This was no accident. The task of delivering daily press conferences had been forced on them by the minister for home affairs. The reason provided was that people needed daily information about the current situation, but it also had the added effect of directing the limelight away from the government — and its withdrawn prime minister.

Now he was staying in the background. While foreign leaders such as the French president, Emmanuel Macron, the prime minister of Denmark, Mette Fredriksen, and Germany's chancellor, Angela Merkel, took over more and more of the efforts to control the virus, the Swedish government let its expert agency make the most important decisions.

On Friday 13 March, the pressure on the government grew. That day, the editor-in-chief of *Dagens Nyheter*, Peter Wolodarski, published an article with the headline 'Close Down Sweden to Protect Sweden'.

Wolodarski argued that Sweden had lost precious time through the Public Health Agency's inaction, and now it was time for the government to take control.

'You can't delegate the decision-making to some state epidemiologist, chief economist, or director-general. In a national crisis, fuelled by an ongoing international crisis, the prime minister must step up, preferably together with the other party leaders, and make open, clear, and effective decisions that inspire confidence and make a real difference.'

In the neighbouring countries, politicians had already steamrolled their expert authorities.

Just seven hours before the Danish prime minister announced her school closures, the head of the Danish Health Authority, Søren Brostrøm, had warned her that the negative consequences would outweigh the positive. And in Norway, the Norwegian Institute of Public Health's director-general, Camilla Stoltenberg, had delivered the same warning to her prime minister.

Would the Swedish government fall into line with its neighbours?

'The world has gone mad'

From his northernly secluded viewpoint, Anders Tegnell could now monitor the course of events unfurling down on the continent.

Norway, Denmark, the Czech Republic, Greece, Austria, Portugal, France — the countries closing their schools and preschools was growing more and more numerous. In the US, 16 states had taken the same measure.

On 14 March, Spain followed Italy's example and went into lockdown. Everyone whose work wasn't essential to society was forced to stay home.

Two days later, the French president, Emmanuel Macron, declared 'war on the virus' and postponed the second round of the country's local elections.

Tegnell couldn't understand what they were doing. To him, it looked as though the other countries were trying to swap out their jet engine mid-flight. Very few of the measures now being implemented were supported by science. Some might even be harmful. Until just a few weeks before, border closures had been considered a wrong turn in the eyes of the public-health sciences. Doctors, drugs, and medical equipment needed to flow freely through the world.

And yet there was a pattern — a kind of logic — in the countries' actions. To understand it, you needed a doctoral degree, not in epidemiology, but in sociology.

A little later that summer, two researchers at Linköping University — Karl Wennberg and Abiel Sebhatu — would show that the measures introduced in different countries were only weakly related to their number of infections, deaths, or available intensive-care beds — things that were standard indicators in epidemiology. A more decisive factor was how many nearby countries had already implemented similar measures.

'Diffusion' — that's what the sociological literature called it when political interventions spread without closer analysis. It was a phenomenon that arose when decisions were made under a great deal of uncertainty.

It was a human thing. Politicians didn't want to be accused of being passive. They wanted to show decisiveness.

But Anders Tegnell wasn't a politician. He was an epidemiologist, and a fairly immovable one at that. He wasn't going to throw out the book of proven tactics. Not over some gut feeling, and not because of peer pressure.

His confidants at the agency agreed with his assessment: the rest of the world was rushing headlong into a dangerous experiment with unforeseen consequences. Lisa Brouwers explained that the Spanish school closures had pushed the virus from the cities to the coasts, as wealthy people fled to their holiday homes. Perhaps that was a reason to keep schools open?

And the Norwegians — what were they thinking? They'd forbidden their citizens from travelling to their second homes, but they were allowed to go to their cabins in Sweden.

'The world has gone mad,' he wrote to Tom Britton and Lisa Brouwers.

It was a phrase that Anders Tegnell would come to repeat throughout the course of the pandemic.

From an epidemiological perspective, Anders Tegnell had a point. A year later, in February 2021, when the Danish parliament presented a report on how Denmark, Norway, Germany, and Sweden had acted around this time, one of the conclusions was that three of the countries had changed course.

'In Denmark, Norway, and Germany, the strategy to combat Covid-19 quickly shifts to make restrictions and bans its main elements. Throughout the entire period, however, Sweden adheres to its strategy based on fewer interventions and informing its citizens,' the investigation stated.

The Swedish strategy now taking shape, thus focused first and foremost on sticking to the plan — to the data, evidence, science — and on not being drawn into what Anders Tegnell saw as madness.

From a human perspective, one might say it was Anders Tegnell who was a bit mad. The easiest option for him personally would no doubt have been to do like everyone else — show cosmetic decisiveness, fall in with Denmark and Norway, and lay low for a bit. No one would blame him in hindsight if he'd been doing like everyone else.

But that wasn't Anders Tegnell's style. And even less Johan Giesecke's.

Giesecke's experience of various dilemmas — like the one now facing the world — was that he was usually right. He felt that way this time, too. On 14 March, he reached out to his old colleagues at the Public Health Agency with an idea.

Giesecke loved diagrams. He had worked with visualisations of numbers almost his entire life, and knew instinctively when the audience would be lost.

Over the years, he'd developed certain opinions about maps (no more than six colours!), he'd arrived at his feelings about three-dimensional pie charts (completely meaningless, *never* use them), and he'd decided that one must always, without exception, explain to the audience what the X and Y axes represent before introducing any other information.

Now Giesecke had a thought: what if the agency drew up a graph of how many people usually died of the flu, and then a line showing the number of Covid deaths in the same frame? That way, people could get a reasonable picture of how harmful — or, rather, harmless — this coronavirus actually was.

The number of deaths due to influenza typically varied a lot from year to year. The worst outbreak in the last few years had been in the winter of 2017–18. That time, around 20,000 Swedes had fallen sick, and 1,012 of them had died.

Giesecke thought the curves should start with the first death, and perhaps be limited to people dying in hospital. This could get both interesting and 'politically' useful.

It ended up being Sweden's deputy state epidemiologist, Anders Wallensten, who replied to Giesecke. By some impractical coincidence, Wallensten had the same first name as the older, ordinary state epidemiologist. Some of the employees at the agency solved this by referring to the 46-year-old — who ran a few dozen miles a week, and always sported a gigantic fitness watch on his wrist — as 'Handsome Anders'.

Handsome Anders was cautiously positive about the idea. Giesecke's diagram might be of pedagogical value. At the same time, wasn't there a risk they might, through such an initiative, be accused of playing down the risks of the new virus?

Nevertheless, Wallensten asked one of the agency's epidemiologists whether there were any influenza figures they could use.

Soon, some investigators and statisticians began to resist Giesecke's idea; it simply wasn't possible to make a fair comparison between Covid-19 and a regular flu. And why would people feel less worried just because the Public Health Agency told them the flu could be an even worse illness?

This irked Johan Giesecke. In his time, lower-level officials hadn't harboured such opinions. Besides, they were wrong.

But there was nothing he could do.

So far, he was just a retired epidemiologist with strong opinions.

Nothing came of the diagram.

* * *

We need to pause here. For if we are to understand Sweden's actions in mid-March 2020 — as well as the actions of the rest of the world — we must first recount two other stories. About a pandemic that took many lives — and one that didn't.

The first story is about the Spanish flu. And yes, it's more than a hundred years old. But unless we delve into it now, it will be impossible to understand how Sweden and the rest of the world came to drift apart.

The year 1918 has been etched into the history of mankind as the year when the Spanish flu began. But we'll be a bit original and start our story in the 1950s, with a Swedish adventurer.

Philadelphia v. St Louis

The first body he found was that of a little girl. Maybe six years old. He had been digging for days. Eighteen hours a day. He had travelled far north in the world to find a place frozen in time.

The year was 1951. The 25-year-old Swedish doctor Johan Hultin harboured a hope that somewhere in the far north there were human bodies, encased in permafrost, in which the virus still lived.

Three decades previously, in 1918, the world's population had been decimated by an influenza that came to be known as the Spanish flu. But a lot remained unknown about the disease. Most of all, no one had found the virus that lay behind this mass death.

Finally, Hultin located a place that might fit the bill.

The village of Brevig Mission, Alaska, had been hit hard by the flu epidemic. Out of 80 inhabitants, 72 had died. When Hultin told the Inuit survivors that he was looking for the virus, he got their permission to dig up the village burial site.

And there he found the little girl. Her black hair had been braided and tied up with bright-red ribbons. Her dress was light grey. Most likely, she'd died in it.

Johan Hultin kept digging. He found more bodies. Using a knife, he cut open their chests, collected lung samples, and placed them in a cooler.

A few days later, he flew home again. Home was no longer Uppsala University but the American Midwest, where he'd got a position as a research student at the University of Iowa.

It took a long time to get back to Iowa. The plane he was travelling in was a propeller-driven DC-3 that kept on having to land to refuel. To keep the samples from being ruined, Hultin had brought along a fire extinguisher, and at every stop he sprayed dry ice over them.

Once back in Iowa City, he tried to inject some of the lung tissue into chicken eggs. He was hoping that the virus would start growing inside them.

But this was 1951. It wasn't just aeroplanes that were inferior back then. These were early days for microbiology, too. Hultin was never successful in his daring experiment.

Nearly half a century later, Johan Hultin read an article in the academic journal *Science*. It was titled 'Initial Genetic Characterization of the 1918 "Spanish" Influenza Virus', and it described how scientists had managed to locate parts of a virus that had killed a 21-year-old soldier in Fort Jackson, South Carolina, in September 1918. Thanks to gene technology, the scientists could determine that the virus was of the type H1N1 — and that it came from pigs and humans.

The letters H and N are a way of describing the influenza virus's genome. H is short for haemagglutinin, and is the 'key' that unlocks human cells and tricks them into producing new viruses. The letter N is short for neuraminidase, which works like a pair of scissors, being used by newly produced virus particles to cut free and infect new cells.

It was a big leap, but a lot remained to figure out.

Johan Hultin thought the time was ripe for another try. Despite having celebrated his 72nd birthday, he decided to return to Alaska — and to foot the bill himself. And this time, he hired helpers for the digging, but brought along a few of his wife's gardening tools so he could take part, too.

The work took five days, and this time it bore better fruit. Six feet below ground, preserved in the permafrost, was the corpse of an overweight Inuit woman. Her lungs were perfectly frozen.

From the woman — whom Hultin called 'Lucy' — it was possible to extract viable genetic material. Together with a third body — from a soldier in his thirties who'd died in New York — scientists were able to present the complete genetic code of the H1N1 virus that had caused the Spanish flu. With the article 'Origin and Evolution of the 1918 "Spanish" Influenza Virus Hemagglutinin Gene' published in 1999, the mystery was solved.

But the final word in the history of the Spanish flu had not yet been written. The virus itself was only half of the story of the disease that claimed an estimated 50 million lives in 1918–19.

Once the microbiological mystery had been solved, the research world turned to studying the politics. How had decision-makers acted?

Could they have done anything differently?

In America, what emerged was a tale of two cities. One was Philadelphia. There, life had largely continued as usual during the late summer of 1918. Larger gatherings had been allowed, including a parade with 200,000 participants to raise money for the great war raging in Europe.

The other city was St Louis. There, doctors had advised local politicians to keep a record of the number of people infected with the flu. And two days after the initial case, schools and churches closed.

The differences between the two cities were stark. In four months, 12,000 Philadelphians died. The excess mortality rate rose to 7,190 people for every one million inhabitants. In St Louis, the corresponding figure was 3,470.

It appeared the politicians' actions in St Louis had saved thousands of lives.

But there might also have been other reasons for the difference in mortality. One of the reasons Philadelphia was hit so hard may have been its location on the east coast. It may also have been the fact that the city lay near two military bases — Fort Dix in New Jersey and Fort Meade in Maryland — and that soldiers who had recently been to Europe fighting in the war were spreading the virus across the city.

This was a piece of history that never seemed to be concluded.

The story about H1N1 wasn't over either. Almost a full century after the Spanish flu, the same virus was able to spread panic in the world once more.

And it would turn into a formative experience for one small country in the north of Europe.

The Mexican sniffles

In the spring of 2009, a Mexican boy called Edgar Hernandez came down with a sudden illness. He lost his appetite, ran a fever, and his body ached all over.

It only took a few days for him to recover, and most likely the whole thing would soon have been forgotten if it weren't for the mucosal test his doctor had sent to a lab in Canada.

When the test came back, it turned out that Edgar had been infected with a new virus — a mix of bird, swine, and human influenza that had blended once more with swine flu. This was a new version of the H1N1 virus, the same one that had once caused the Spanish flu.

The five-year-old from Mexico became world-famous in an instant. Fear of the 'Mexican flu', or the 'swine flu' as it would later be known, spread across the world.

Panic spread, too. Birds were slaughtered in Hong Kong, pigs were killed in Egypt, one German state advised its citizens not to kiss.

In Sweden, the major tabloid *Aftonbladet* published a story about a man watching TV in his home when he suddenly fell sick. 'By the time the ambulance arrived, he was already dead,' it said in the text, which was given the headline: '37-year-old Died Within a Few Hours'.

It was the first death in Sweden from the virus. Few cared about the fact that the man had also suffered from an underlying condition.

It wasn't the first time the papers and TV stations of the world had whipped up a pandemic threat. A mere three years earlier, it had been a bird flu spreading terror.

But this time was different, in more ways than one. Most of all, the monitoring systems had been expanded. Viruses that wouldn't have been discovered in the past could now be found and categorised. More than 130 laboratories in 102 countries worked tirelessly to identify new strains of influenza. Some doctors and epidemiologists quietly began to joke that 'WHO' was short for 'World Hysteria Organization'.

Another factor was the increasing influence of scientific data models. Estimates of between 2 and 7.4 million deaths were mentioned — and those were calculations based on a mild pandemic. If the virus turned out to be as aggressive as the H1N1 virus that had caused the Spanish flu, the global death toll would be in the tens of millions.

But most of all, the commotion surrounding previous pandemics had generated political decisions. One such decision, made by the Social Democratic government after the 2006 avian flu, was to task the National Board of Health and Welfare with drawing up agreements to secure Sweden's access to a vaccine in case of a pandemic.

The following year, a contract was signed with GlaxoSmithKline. It meant that Sweden would get priority access to a vaccine — but also that the National Board of Health and Welfare bound itself to certain commitments. If the WHO classed an influenza outbreak as a full-on pandemic, the board would have ten days to determine how many doses the country needed.

The WHO hadn't classified a disease as a full-scale pandemic in 40 years. Formally, such a decision would mean that the risk classification was raised to six on a scale from one to six.

Neither were the definitions entirely clear. In some WHO documents, a pandemic meant an 'enormous number of deaths', while formal regulations referred to an uncontrolled spread of a new virus. Moreover, individual countries could, to some extent, do as they liked. The United Kingdom classed the swine flu as a pandemic early on — as early as 1 May 2009.

On 11 June 2009 came the decision from the WHO. The swine flu had been raised to level six.

At this time, Anders Tegnell was head of the unit for infectious-disease control at the National Board of Health and Welfare. When the decision came from the WHO, it triggered a formal process. He was now bound by the contracts that had been signed. If he didn't do anything, Sweden would automatically get 18 million doses of the vaccine, which had been given the name Pandemrix. At the same time, doctors around the country were advising him not to buy the vaccine. There was much evidence to indicate that Sweden was experiencing only a mild variant of the virus.

In the middle of the night, Anders Tegnell emailed his friend Johan Carlson.

What should they do? He explained that the message from the government had been that there was 'no turning back'. By then, Carlson had become the director-general of the Swedish Institute for Infectious Disease Control — the government agency that would later turn into the Public Health Agency of Sweden.

He replied: 'Infectious-disease doctors have to realise that this is business and politics rather than medicine.'

Most other countries chose to wait. In Denmark, only at-risk groups were vaccinated. In Poland, the health minister, Ewa Kopacz, claimed there was a conflict of interest between drug companies and public health. Despite being subjected to harsh criticism from other politicians in her country, she chose not to buy a single dose.

Lisa Brouwers, at this time working as a researcher at the Institute for Infectious Disease Control, was calculating the socio-economic consequences of a mass vaccination.

She erred on the side of caution. She assumed a low R_0 of 1.4, and a relatively low risk of dying — around five deaths per every 100,000 infections.

Nevertheless, the answer was clear.

When the computers finished crunching the data, they revealed that society would save 2.5 billion SEK if at least 60 per cent of the population got the vaccine. But even at a 30 per cent vaccination rate, it would pay off.

What made it look so good were the absent costs of sick leave, doctor visits, days spent home with sick children, and hospital stays. The price tag for each life saved had been set at 22 million SEK; but even excluding that, the vaccination was profitable.

Sweden ended up buying 18 million doses — two for every citizen — at a cost of 1.3 billion SEK. In October 2009, a mass vaccination of the Swedish people was initiated. It was completely voluntary, but the Swedes trusted their authorities. A total of 5.3 million Swedes were vaccinated — a higher proportion than in any other country.

But a year later, another cost would arise. In August 2010 came the first reports of an increased frequency of the neurological condition known as narcolepsy among children and young people vaccinated with Pandemrix.

The cases kept growing. Now, ten years later, more than 400 people had been awarded compensation by the Swedish Pharmaceutical Insurance organisation. They had all been struck by sudden attacks of narcolepsy, and hallucinations, or one of the other symptoms brought on by the condition.

Knowing this in hindsight, Anders Tegnell would still believe that he'd done the right thing at the time — he'd made his decision based on the knowledge available to him. Indeed, it would even have been unethical not to buy those doses, he would say to anyone who asked.

It was a simple calculation. The public-health authorities assumed that about a hundred lives would be saved by the mass vaccination. They didn't know the risks. In a way, he said to *Dagens Nyheter*, they were lucky they didn't know about the side effects. If so, they would have had to weigh the risk of narcolepsy against the expected deaths from swine flu. Once again: the state's calculation wasn't the same as that of the individual.

In 2009, Johan Giesecke followed the whole thing from a distance. He was sitting just a stone's throw from the Institute for Infectious Disease Control, now as chief scientist at the newly formed European Centre for Disease Prevention and Control in Solna. He was, for once, disconnected from Swedish decision-making. But Brouwer's investigation had been published in the ECDC's own journal, *Eurosurveillance*, and Giesecke himself had appeared on Sweden's Television stating that, as far as they knew, the vaccine was less dangerous than the flu itself.

Many older infectious-disease patriarchs were strongly critical of Tegnell and Carlson. Lars Olof Kallings, who had formerly been head of the National Bacteriological Laboratory, thought everyone involved had lost their heads. He wrote a book in which he referred to the swine flu as 'the Mexican sniffles', and accused the drug companies of defrauding the entire world. The WHO couldn't be trusted anymore. Their decisions were 'not always medically motivated'.

Even though Anders Tegnell would defend his decision for all eternity, the swine flu incident left its mark on Swedish society. The decision-making process became the subject of political science essays, journalists shone a light on the WHO's connections to the pharmaceutical industry, and the media panic was dissected after the fact. *Svenska Dagbladet*, the newspaper that had issued the loudest warnings against the risks of the vaccine, published some conspicuous we-told-you-so editorials: 'A looming, deadly world epidemic with powerful, dramatic images constitutes an almost irresistible cocktail for newspapers. They get going and egg each other on, and the hunt is led by news editors whose medical knowledge is most often hazy,' wrote *Svenska Dagbladet*'s medical reporter, Inger Atterstam.

Three years after the pandemic, *Svenska Dagbladet* was able to reveal new calculations by Lisa Brouwers. They showed that only six human lives had been saved by the mass vaccination. As more and more cases of narcolepsy were discovered, the figures looked worse and worse.

Those responsible turned even more inward. Johan Giesecke only replied to questions via email, and the then head of information at the Institute for Infectious Disease Control, Aase Sten, sent out talking points for everyone to stick to: do compare with Norway and Finland, which have more deaths; don't compare with Poland; generally, we know very little about lives saved; the best strategy for Sweden was to vaccinate the entire population. Et cetera.

But it was one thing to defend their line of action externally. It was another to believe in it.

The Swedish Strategy

Eleven years later, Sweden chose a path that deviated from the rest of the world once more. And just like during the swine flu, Sweden now followed a plan whose central components had in fact been decided long before.

In 2009, Anders Tegnell had upheld the vaccine agreements. And now, in March 2020, he upheld the pandemic plan that had been renewed just a few months earlier, in November 2019.

After making the rounds within both the Public Health Agency and the government, the Swedish strategy was formulated in 35 words and later published on the government's website: 'The overall objective of the government's efforts is to reduce the pace of the Covid-19 virus's spread: to "flatten the curve" so that large numbers of people do not become ill at the same time.'

Initially, that sentence was fairly uncontroversial. 'Flattening the curve' had long been an established concept in public health. According to epidemiological mythology, the American doctor Howard Markel had come up with the phrase in Atlanta in 2007. He'd ordered Thai food, opened the box, and noticed that his dinner was a flattened block of noodles instead of an appetising little mound.

But during a few days in mid-March, when several European countries seemed to spare no expense in clamping down on the new virus, certain parts of the Swedish strategy began to stand out. These were, partly, the approach that measures ought to 'be weighed against their effects on society and public health in general' and, partly, formulations about *reducing the pace* and avoiding a lot of people *becoming ill at the same time.*

Sweden, too, introduced restrictions. But they were cautious, and followed the laid-out strategy. On 11 March — the same day that the first death was recorded in the country, that the WHO officially declared Covid-19 a pandemic, and that larger gatherings were banned in Sweden — the government scrapped a rule in the national health insurance scheme that had meant you didn't get paid for your first day of sick leave.

A few days later, people over the age of 70 were advised to limit their contact with others as much as possible. The next day, upper-secondary schools and universities were encouraged to teach remotely. The government also recommended that Swedes not visit nursing homes. Several municipalities and aged-care companies went further, introducing blanket bans on visits.

Anders Tegnell thought one positive side effect of the Swedish strategy was that many of the little details scientists squabbled over weren't so important. For example, whether asymptomatic transmission actually occurred didn't matter hugely, as Sweden's goal wasn't to avoid every instance of transmission.

What about children, could they be contagious? If so, not very. But were some children contagious? If so, they weren't a big source of transmission. The idea was to grapple with larger amounts of transmission — to *reduce the pace*, not *reduce at any cost*.

On Thursday 12 March, Anders Tegnell stood in Sweden's Television's studio, listening to an interview with Maurizio Grosso.

Grosso was a doctor in Italy, and he was sharing his experience of the situation. He felt that it was reminiscent of the Second World War — of the bombing of Rimini. Young people were dying, too, he said. People without underlying health conditions. The segment was illustrated with scenes that could have been picked out of a disaster film: cleaners in protective clothing decontaminating the streets.

Grosso had one piece of advice for the Swedes: close schools, theatres, and museums.

Anders Tegnell had no such plans. The research gave no support to the suggestion that closing down society would be a better measure than the ones Sweden had already implemented.

His appearance was part of what he and Jan Albert were calling a 'campaign for understanding'. As panic now spread through the world, it was important to stand your ground, to put things in their true perspective.

The way he saw it, it wasn't rational to deal with small amounts of infection that wouldn't cause large-scale transmission in society.

Tegnell felt good about the Swedish line. In truth, what he'd written to Britton and Brouwers about the world going mad was a bit of an exaggeration. There were still countries following their old plans. Especially hopeful was the fact that the British were yet to get swept up in the hysteria.

But this was an entirely new situation. Not one of the tens of thousands of epidemiologists, mathematicians, microbiologists, economists, political scientists, and virologists now putting all their other research on hold had experienced anything like this before: a new virus spreading across the globe through what appeared to be a completely susceptible population.

There were no answers. There were only more or less well-founded hypotheses.

The Swedes shaping the country's strategy — formally and informally — would now make a number of assumptions that deviated radically from those made in the rest of the world.

A little dirt is good for you

In March 2020, countries around the world began to keep meticulous statistics of the number of positive viral tests. Online traffic to sites such as Worldometer — reporting the figures for each country and administrative region — increased by the day.

The fight against the spread of the virus was visualised in line graphs and bars. They were like stock charts, only inverted. Up was bad; down was good.

But within epidemiology — at least, such as the science had been up until a few months prior — it wasn't so simple. Decreased transmission of a virus was not always a good thing.

The classic example was rubella. It was a disease caused by the rubella virus, and up until the 1970s was one of the most common childhood illnesses in Sweden.

The term 'childhood illness' is really quite misleading. Infectious diseases belonging to this group — including whooping cough, mumps, and chickenpox — can afflict anyone. But as they are highly contagious and yield lifelong immunity, few adults are ever affected.

For adults who did get rubella, it usually wasn't that bad. The disease could cause itching and sometimes enlarged lymph nodes, but it would pass.

The problems arose if a pregnant woman was infected with rubella. There was a substantial risk that she might miscarry, or give birth to a child with deformities of the skeleton, brain, or eyes.

The rubella epidemic that raged in the US between 1962 and 1964 is estimated to have harmed 20,000 children.

There were thus multiple reasons to attempt to eradicate the disease.

But it was more complicated than many thought.

In the mid-1970s, Greek one-year-olds started being vaccinated against rubella. The main purpose wasn't to prevent them from having to go through the disease as young children, but to protect them later in life. However, when almost 20 years had passed, something unexpected happened. It turned out that the number of rubella cases in young adults was higher than ever since 1950.

Despite nearly half of all one-year-olds getting vaccinated for two decades, young women were running an even greater risk of catching the infection while pregnant.

What had happened?

Soon, scientists discovered that the cause was the vaccination program itself.

Previously — before the 1970s — a Greek four- or five-year-old who hadn't yet been infected had a good chance of picking up the virus from a younger sibling, or perhaps from a schoolmate with siblings at home. But as younger children were vaccinated, their exposure decreased. There was thus a large group of people running a substantially lower risk — or, rather, with a lower chance — of getting their dose of the disease as children. Nor had they received the vaccine.

Twenty years later, the effect became visible.

In the literature that many future infectious-disease doctors and epidemiologists had to study, certain conclusions were drawn from the Greek example. One seminal work was titled *Modern Infectious Disease Epidemiology*. It had been printed in several editions, and the author of the book — Giesecke — advised the world's agencies for infectious-disease control not to initiate a vaccination program for rubella unless herd immunity could be guaranteed.

The instance in Greece wasn't the only case of a measure designed to prevent an infectious disease from having unforeseen consequences. When, around the same time, a number of European countries suffered deaths linked to listeriosis, several scientists concluded that it was — paradoxically — caused by improved hygiene in the food industry.

Listeriosis was caused by listeria, a common bacterium living in soil and water. If it ended up in food, it could spread to humans. If young people became infected, they were sometimes asymptomatic, and sometimes got what appeared to be a very mild cold or stomach bug.

It was worse for frail people — the elderly, and people with multiple diagnoses — and newborns were hit harder. And for pregnant women it could lead to miscarriage or premature birth. For this reason, government agencies in several countries thought at-risk groups should avoid everything from unpasteurised dairy products, medium-rare steaks, and mouldy cheese, to gravlax.

The recommendations varied across different countries. But this wasn't the advice scientists were targeting. The larger problem was that such a big part of the food that humans consumed nowadays was free from certain bacteria.

For when their exposure to listeria decreased, many people avoided infection early in life. And because the bacterium hadn't been fully eradicated, they ran the risk of being badly affected when they were older and more vulnerable.

This was related to what was known as the 'hygiene hypothesis'. It had been formulated in 1989 by the scientist David Strachan: in short, its main idea was that germs make our immune system stronger, while excessive cleanliness makes us less healthy.

Pretty much every language in the world has an equivalent to the Swedish expression 'a little dirt will clean out your tummy'. Back in the day in the US and the UK, old men and women could say: 'You'll eat a peck of dirt before you die.'

With Strachan's hygiene hypothesis, that attitude had been transformed from folklore into modern science. Excessive cleanliness was singled out as the cause behind eczema and allergies. It turned out that those who had grown up in the countryside, with parents who were farmers and thus in closer contact with animals, were afflicted by certain ailments to a much lower extent.

Prominent doctors in immunology now encouraged people to expose their children to peanuts, and to throw out anti-bacterial cleaning products. When the Pulitzer Prize–winning *New York Times* journalist Matt Richtel published a book about the immune system titled *An Elegant Defense*, he summarised the findings with the suggestion: 'So maybe you should pick your nose and eat what you extract?'

Maybe; maybe not. The jury was still out on that one. But one thing was increasingly clear. Study after study was produced on how we'd upset a delicate balance. For thousands of years — millions of years, if you counted the time before we were humans — our immune system had been under constant attack. Now, it had less to do.

While science uncovered the dirty secret, society was moving in the opposite direction. We cleaned our homes as though they were operating theatres. A small bottle of hand sanitiser could be found in each man and woman's accessories.

But among the older generation, folk wisdom lived on. And so perhaps it was no accident that it was an older person who, on 14 March 2020, planted the idea in the state epidemiologist's mind.

That day, a 78-year-old woman from the south of Sweden got in touch with Anders Tegnell. She had long been retired, but had once worked as an oncologist in Lund. She'd conducted some research, too.

The situation had become completely hysterical, she now felt. Why couldn't they just do what people did back in the day?

She described how it used to work. If one boy got chickenpox, no one would isolate him. Quite the opposite. All the neighbours would send their kids over, so they could get the illness, too.

Chickenpox worked the same way as rubella. It was pretty much harmless to have as a child, but a lot worse as an adult.

If it was like Tegnell said on TV — that younger adults and children only experienced mild symptoms — why didn't they just rent a bunch of hotels where they could send people who wanted to get infected? It could be voluntary, and these days the hotels were empty anyway. Then you'd have a large group of citizens who could work freely, study freely, and perhaps take care of others.

It wasn't the first time Anders Tegnell heard a version of that idea. One of the people who were cautiously positive about letting the lives of younger Swedes go on as usual was Johan Giesecke. After all, the Anthroposophists in Järna — those people refusing to get vaccinated — even had measles parties. Though that might be a bit much, Giesecke thought. After all, a fair amount of people got really quite sick from the measles.

Nevertheless, it was an idea.

Anders Tegnell sent off an email about the 78-year-old doctor's thoughts to his Finnish colleague Mika Salminen.

Salminen was the director of the Institute for Health and Welfare in Finland, and somewhat like Tegnell's equivalent across the Baltic.

Tegnell had no plans to rent a few thousand hotel rooms at Scandic or Best Western, but he thought the logic lent support to keeping schools open: 'One point would support keeping schools open to quicker reach herd immunity.'

Salminen replied that they had considered it, too, but children would still be able to spread the infection while they were sick.

'True, but probably mostly to each other,' Tegnell wrote back.

The reason for this was that younger Swedes didn't tend to live with older Swedes. Unlike in southern European countries, very few families had a grandmother living upstairs.

Mika Salminen explained that his modellers had calculated that one in every 10 cases of illness among the elderly could be avoided if schools stayed open.

Anders Tegnell thought that sounded good. Ten per cent, you say? He suggested that the Swedish and Finnish numbers people get together for a meeting.

'It might be worth it,' Tegnell wrote.

'A tsunami of a relatively mild disease'

'One minus one over R_0. It's in my book.'

Johan Giesecke liked to refer to the equation explaining how many Swedes would have to be infected before that magic kicked in — the one that Ross, Topley, Hedrich, and the others had spent a century figuring out.

In digits: $1-(1/R_0)$.

The final piece of the puzzle — the equation itself — had been solved by C.E.G. Smith and K. Dietz in the 1970s. What it meant was that the more contagious a disease is, the harder it becomes to reach herd immunity. If the value of R_0 is high, the denominator below the second figure one becomes bigger.

Let's say we invent an extremely contagious virus with an R_0 of 100. Such a disease would have a herd-immunity threshold of $1-(1/100)$.

That is: 99/100, or 99 per cent.

In the middle of March 2020, most scientists believed the coronavirus had an R_0 of somewhere between 2 and 3. This was relatively high: for the coronavirus known as MERS discovered in Saudi Arabia in 2012, R_0 had been estimated as somewhere between 0.8 and 1.3.

This new coronavirus was different; it was more contagious and a lot less deadly than both MERS and SARS.

If R_0 for the novel coronavirus was 2, it meant that more than half of all Swedes would have to be infected before herd immunity could arise.

That seemed difficult.

But Johan Giesecke saw the situation differently. If the virus spread so quickly, it meant the pandemic would soon be over. It also meant the restrictions introduced by all those other countries would turn out to be useless.

He searched for a metaphor. Perhaps the virus was like a tidal wave? A tsunami?

Yes, a tsunami. You can protect yourself from it, climb up on a roof, flee up a mountain, but you can't stop it.

'A tsunami of a relatively mild disease.' That's how he began to speak of the new coronavirus.

To those who sought his expertise — the group at the WHO, a Swedish pension fund manager, journalists, the Public Health Agency — he said that several of the world's countries were now painting themselves into a corner. If they closed down because of a virus that would return as soon as restrictions eased, when would they be able to open up again? What level of transmission would they have to accept?

Would they maintain school closures and limited mobility until there was a vaccine? How long would that be?

The only way to solve this was by letting the virus spread at a controlled rate until it had nowhere to go. That was how influenza epidemics ended.

Much later, this would come to be known as a herd-immunity strategy. But to Johan Giesecke, it wasn't a strategy so much as a scientific fact.

This was just the way it was.

The third option

Far out on the Baltic Sea, in an easterly bay of Gotland, an island that was always deserted in winter, Peet Tüll followed the spread of the virus from inside a white stucco house with red window casings.

Early in the morning on 15 March, he sat down in front of his computer and started typing an email to Anders Tegnell.

They had known each other for a long time. Twenty-five years earlier, Tüll had received a request from the WHO for assistance during an Ebola outbreak in the city of Kikwit, Zaire, in 1995. No one in Sweden really understood what the WHO wanted, so Tüll thought he might as well send two doctors right away.

One of them was Anders Tegnell.

Peet Tüll had initially been head of the infectious-disease clinic in Visby, the only big town on the island, and then head of the unit for infectious-disease control at the National Board of Health and Welfare. Many of his tasks would later be baked into the state epidemiologist position.

In that post, Tüll had been part of developing the *Communicable Diseases Act* passed by parliament in 2004. He liked to say that he'd written the law himself. About this, Johan Giesecke said that it was a typical Peet Tüll thing to say; but, sure, it was true.

At any rate, when Peet Tüll retired, Anders Tegnell was the one who took over his job. At the same time, the job description was expanded, and the position was later absorbed by the newly formed Public Health Agency.

But in some sense it was Anders Tegnell's predecessor who emailed him that Sunday morning in March.

'Hi Anders. There are three strategies for stopping the pandemic,' Peet Tüll wrote.

The first option was a total shutdown of society for four weeks. The second option was to locate as many infected people as possible, tracing all close contacts, and putting them under a two-week quarantine. The third option: 'Letting the virus spread, slow or fast, to reach a hypothetical "herd immunity".'

Peet Tüll advocated option two. Sweden was still in an advantageous position, with few infections and few deaths.

Choosing option three, however, would lead to thousands of deaths.

'It seems to me a defeatist and headless strategy, which I would never have accepted in my previous role.'

A few hours later, in the early afternoon, Tegnell replied: 'Yes, we have trudged through this and nevertheless arrived at number three. We probably have fairly extensive transmission, which would mean the first two won't work.'

That weekend, the term for herd immunity — *flockimmunitet* — would be transformed from an obscure technical term into one of the most loaded words in the Swedish language.

Because the same day that Tüll and Tegnell were emailing each other in confidence, another doctor was putting the finishing touches to her Kremlinological analysis of what the Public Health Agency was up to.

At 72 years of age, Annika Linde was about the same age as many of the men who both devised and criticised the Swedish strategy. She had been an infectious-disease doctor, then a researcher at the department for viruses at the former National Bacteriological Laboratory. Eventually, she became one of the world's foremost experts on influenza.

In 2005, she was appointed as state epidemiologist — after Johan Giesecke.

Giesecke wasn't entirely happy about the choice of his successor. He and Linde had bickered quite a bit during management meetings at the Institute for Infectious Disease Control, 'like an old married couple', he said. And he would have preferred to see an epidemiologist — not a virologist — getting the job.

'But seeing as we are running low on epidemiologists in Sweden, Annika is a good choice,' he'd said to the medical trade publication *Dagens Medicin,* in what can be translated as a half-blessing.

Annika Linde stayed in the job until 2013, when she was succeeded by Anders Tegnell.

In other words, she had a somewhat unique insight into the thinking of Swedish epidemiologists in general. And on Sunday 15 March, she shared it with the world.

In a long Facebook post, she described what herd immunity meant: those who had not been infected were protected by the big immune herd.

'If we could reach herd immunity here, with as little transmission as possible to sensitive risk groups, we could minimise the economic as well as medical consequences of the Covid to a high degree.'

So far, the damage wasn't that bad. But soon the text would turn into a PR disaster for the Public Health Agency.

It started when she quoted a proverb from the early 20th century: 'Influenza is the old man's friend.'

'People already at the end of life were nudged over the edge, and drifted away into the carbon-dioxide narcosis that sets in (after a period of suffering) when you're not breathing properly. That's not our reasoning today. We want to be able to save an elderly person or someone with multiple diagnoses enjoying their life. Doing that requires qualified hospital care, and if so, chaos will ensue within the healthcare services if we let the virus loose completely.'

She continued: 'But, as there is no vaccine, I would still like for us to keep a moderate level of transmission going among younger people, with herd immunity as our goal.'

And her conclusion: 'What I have described is in fact our Public Health Agency's strategy. I see it as the best possible in a pretty impossible situation!'

The former state epidemiologist's post became big news. That same day, the TT News Agency published a text with the headline 'Controversial Strategy May Save Lives', which it cabled to newspapers all over the country.

For a text written by a news agency, it was uncharacteristically evocative: 'The time to stop the virus has passed, and epidemiologists are increasingly coming to understand that this virus is here to stay. It won't let up until a majority of Swedes have been infected,' read the closing lines.

Peet Tüll had a completely different view of what a herd-immunity approach would entail. While darkness fell over Gotland that Sunday, he continued to email back and forth with Anders Tegnell.

Tegnell wrote to him that options 1 and 2 probably wouldn't work as Sweden most likely had 'extensive silent transmission'.

'It's worked in China and South Korea,' Tüll wrote. 'So there is no reason why it wouldn't work here?'

Their conversation quickly turned both technical and aggressive. Tüll asked more questions. Had the National Board of Health and Welfare issued general advice or regulations? What was the Health and Social Care Inspectorate doing? Was it following up to ensure sufficient resources? If there was a lack of reagents for testing, couldn't the Public Health Agency ask China or South Korea?

Tegnell replied curtly, in an email lacking both punctuation and a preposition: 'Didn't work Italy doesn't seem to be working in other EU countries either

The answer to most of the other questions is no'

There was nothing Tüll could do to make Tegnell change his mind. In one final email, which received no reply from Tegnell, he wrote: 'The conditions in Italy are completely different from Sweden. You can't just stand idly by if you fear a large number of people might die. Any possibility to prevent it from happening must be seized. It isn't enough to "believe" that it's not possible.'

Peet Tüll and Annika Linde weren't the only doctors airing their thoughts that weekend. That same Sunday, *Svenska Dagbladet*'s culture section published a piece by Johan von Schreeb about Peter Wolodarski. In two Sunday columns in a row, the editor-in-chief of *Dagens Nyheter* had criticised both the Public Health Agency and the government.

In his piece, the famous doctor now berated Wolodarski for questioning 'existing knowledge, research, and expertise' in 'polarising language and with a basis in exceedingly vague evidence'.

Johan von Schreeb thought Wolodarski's opinions were peculiar. In one of his articles, Wolodarski had held up Israel as a model. Israel, von Schreeb asked. Their lockdown was based on politics — not infectious-disease control. This was a country where security was a political product, where external threats functioned as a cohesive glue holding society together.

Johan von Schreeb had emailed Wolodarski and asked him to back off. He had received no response. So now he was writing an op-ed instead.

'Disavowing on such weak grounds an all-but-unified Swedish expertise, which has spent decades building up a reliable store of knowledge, is both terrifying and disconcerting.'

Johan von Schreeb linked Wolodarski's behaviour to the contempt for knowledge, research, and expertise that had been unfurling across the rest of the world in the last few years.

'I see it in the US, in Hungary, in Russia, and never have I seen it as clearly in Sweden as now.'

It was an interesting role reversal for von Schreeb. Only nine days before, he had been one of the three doctors on a pilgrimage to the Public Health Agency to warn Anders Tegnell of the new virus.

Now he was coming to the state epidemiologist's defence.

'Should we let politics and fear rule,' he asked, 'over the knowledge and experience among the officials who have been working with infectious-disease control and outbreaks for decades?'

The question was meant to be rhetorical. But for politicians around the world, it was now becoming exceedingly real and concrete.

'Go England!'

The following day, on Monday 16 March, Anders Tegnell watched an eight-minute YouTube clip.

'Good afternoon, everybody,' said a man with a bad haircut.

The man was wearing a suit and a spotted tie, and spoke in way that didn't reveal where among the British Isles he'd grown up, but — on the other hand — did reveal which social class he belonged to. This was the speech of a man who'd gone to a public school.

'We have a clear plan that we are now working through.'

The name of the man on the screen was Boris Johnson and, as of eight months ago, he was the prime minister of the United Kingdom.

'And we're now getting onto the next phase in that plan.'

After a few minutes, Boris Johnson handed over to Sir Patrick Vallance, the British government's chief scientific adviser, who explained that they had identified 590 cases in the country, but between 5,000 and 10,000 people had likely been infected.

The government was now trying to flatten the curve of infections and push it further into the future — preferably into the summer, when the healthcare system was generally under less strain.

To achieve this, they had an entire battery of measures: a blanket quarantine if even one member of your household got infected, bans on large gatherings, and so on.

'But if you do that at the moment, you're not protecting anybody, really, because the number of cases is too small,' Vallance said.

If restrictions were introduced too soon, there was also a risk that families might have to go into quarantine multiple times.

'But it's important to realise that it's not a matter of preventing everyone from getting the virus. That's not possible. Neither is it desirable, as we want some level of immunity in the population. We need immunity to protect us against this in the future,' Vallance said.

The video was actually four days old. It was from a press conference on 12 March. But Jan Albert had sent it to Tegnell that morning.

Tegnell wasn't the only one who received it. Albert had sent the same clip to Johan Giesecke, Anders Wallensten, Johan von Schreeb, and several others. In the subject line, he'd written: 'Go England!'

'Take a look at this press conference with Boris Johnson and their state epidemiologists. Especially when the latter come in after ca 8 min. Good stuff!'

Really, there wasn't a whole lot new being said. Everything Boris Johnson and Patrick Vallance accounted for was standard pandemic management: first a phase of contact tracing — which was now over — and then a phase of damage control.

But they no doubt possessed an eloquence that few other government officials in the world could boast of.

It impressed Tegnell.

'Wonderful, isn't it,' he replied.

The last person speaking in the YouTube clip was Chris Whitty, England's chief medical officer. He explained another thought behind the strategy: 'If people start too soon, they'll get very tired.'

What he meant was that people's patience with restrictions was limited. After a while they'd grow weary, perhaps ignore the advice, and the impact would be lower than it could have been.

This phenomenon came to be known as 'behavioural fatigue', but as yet there was no scientific support for the belief that people would eventually get fed up with restrictions.

It wasn't so strange. After all, the restrictions now being introduced or planned in several countries had never been tested on a grand scale before.

Anders Tegnell believed in the phenomenon, too. It would even form a small puzzle piece in the Swedish strategy. The fact that there were no scientific studies supporting the belief was of less significance. Anyone could see that you could only restrict people's lives so much and for so long.

'I don't think you need science to back that up. Shutting down society completely won't work. There's no need for big studies on that,' he said.

Sometimes you just had to go with your gut.

What neither Jan Albert nor Anders Tegnell knew that morning, as they admired the British decision-makers' ability to present a short and concise outline of their pandemic strategy, was that this strategy was already about to shift.

Soon, the UK would change tack.

And Sweden would be all alone in the world.

Part III

Professor Lockdown

The same day Anders Tegnell and his colleagues watched the video clip, a report was made public in the UK. It had not yet been peer-reviewed, but its 20 pages would come to have a big impact on how the world dealt with the new virus.

The name of its main author was Neil Ferguson. He was a lean 51-year-old with glasses and the same sense of fashion as Anders Tegnell, if perhaps with a slightly more urban twist. Instead of Tegnell's polo shirt, corduroys, and boat shoes, he wore jeans, a T-shirt, and a sports coat.

People said Ferguson was both a workaholic and an exercise junkie. He kept himself up to date on technical details and basic research, all the while taking on more and more managerial duties. In his office at Imperial College was a treadmill that, to his great dismay, couldn't be sped up to more than a few miles per hour.

Despite — or because of — this industriousness, he was appreciated by his younger colleagues. He'd solve small, technical problems for them, and when he received an appreciative email from some dignitary he'd reply and ask the sender to rephrase the message, directing their praise to all of his colleagues so he could forward it to his entire research team.

On the list of Neil Ferguson's merits were several publications in prestigious journals. Among other places, his name appeared in the eight-page study in *The Lancet* about school closures co-authored by Anders Tegnell.

The report that Neil Ferguson presented at 5.00 pm on Monday 16 March had been making the rounds for a while in London and Washington. Boris Johnson's government had seen it, and two days previously the White House had received a draft.

But that afternoon, it was brought to the public's attention.

On page eight of the report was a chart illustrating the damage the virus would cause in society. Wave-shaped curves in different colours showed how many intensive-care beds would be needed in different scenarios. And at the bottom — barely noticeable — was a red line showing how many such beds existed in the country.

It was a statistical bloodbath for the UK. If nothing was done, almost a quarter of a million intensive-care beds could be required — thirty times more than the country had.

But the politicians had a choice. They could decide on what were known as 'non-pharmaceutical interventions' that would reduce the rate of transmission in various ways, pushing that R_0 number down.

The measures presented, each in a different colour, were options such as closing schools and universities, isolating those infected, and introducing various quarantine rules.

With every measure, the strain on the healthcare services eased a little. In the best-case scenario, only a third as many hospital beds would be needed, compared with nothing being done.

The British government's strategy, which had been repeated by its chief scientific adviser, Patrick Vallance, in an interview with the BBC as recently as three days prior, now appeared heartless. Simply letting the virus spread freely would, according to Ferguson's investigations, result in 510,000 British deaths.

There was a calculation pertaining to the US as well, according to which political passivity could result in 2.2 million American deaths.

Ferguson's report grew wings. Its charts were reproduced by media outlets around the world, its figures reshuffled and applied by scientists in other countries. With Ferguson's model, each country could forecast how many would die. It would be cited by government representatives in Germany and France; a few days later, the UK would initiate an extensive lockdown of society; and two weeks after its presentation, the US president, Donald Trump, would stand in front of a chart based on Ferguson's calculations.

In a short time, everything changed. Neil Ferguson was declared a hero in the UK and given the epithet 'Professor Lockdown'.

But two days later, Johan Giesecke got a new job.

And he was less than impressed.

'Fortune tellers and magicians'

'Who names a university Imperial College? The college of the *empire*? How does that sound? How very British — they sure think highly of themselves.'.

As Neil Ferguson presented his report, Johan Giesecke stepped back into the government agency where he'd once served as the state epidemiologist. It may have changed its name — from the Swedish Institute for Infectious Disease Control to the Public Health Agency of Sweden — and got some additional tasks to fulfil, but in all respects it was a triumphant return for the 70-year-old man who, according to the agency's own guidelines, should have been off isolating somewhere.

'They've dusted me off!' he said cheerfully.

It was Anders Tegnell who had asked him in a brief email if he wanted to come in and do some work. Giesecke had replied 'Why not?', and now here he was, with an access pass in his pocket and a sparkle in his eye.

The open-plan office was a bit strange, he thought. But at least the coffee in the cafeteria was free nowadays.

Anders Tegnell and Johan Giesecke. Together again. Only this time in reversed roles.

Unlike the time when Giesecke had given Tegnell a job, the former received a very clear assignment from Tegnell: his role was to go through the advanced scientific models of transmission and death spinning around the world.

But the thing was, Giesecke wasn't particularly fond of more complex models. Sure, he wrote about them in his books, and he commented on their underlying equations. But the forecasts that turned out to be wrong were almost more interesting. They spoke more about what the world really looked like.

One such forecast, the figures of which he knew like an old phone number and liked to refer to, was about mad cow disease. Two decades previously, in 2001, the British had slaughtered roughly four million livestock to prevent the disease from spreading.

'They thought 50,000 people would die. So how many did?'

He answered his own question.

'One hundred and seventy-seven.'

Then a brief pause for effect.

'Not 177,000. One hundred and seventy-seven.'

He had more examples. Four years later, Imperial College warned that 150 million people around the world might die of bird flu. It ended up being 455. Four years after that, it was swine flu. That time, the prognosis forecast 65,000 British deaths. The results? Four hundred and seventy-four.

Why would anyone trust the British scientists now?

Johan Giesecke knew Neil Ferguson well. The world's epidemiological elite consisted of some 100 people, and he'd met everyone in it — at conferences, within the WHO, and at meetings between epidemiologists in different parts of the world.

The epidemiologists of the world functioned as a kind of parallel diplomatic corps. Countries sent their representatives out into the world to discover threats and dangers early on, to be part of committees tied to the UN or the EU — but also to build networks and informal connections that could be activated in a crisis.

It was a small world.

Now, Neil Ferguson hadn't named Imperial College himself. But Giesecke thought its name had quite a bit in common with Ferguson's personality.

'He can be rather superior. Englishmen can be a bit arrogant. Sometimes they come across as thinking they're a little better than everyone else. Not a lot better, just a tiny bit better.'

When Johan Giesecke spoke of Imperial College, it could sometimes sound as if he were describing a family feud in southern Italy that had gone on for generations and whose vendettas had been inherited down the ages.

And if Giesecke was the patriarch of Swedish epidemiology, the name of his equivalent in the UK was Roy Anderson.

Sir Roy, as Giesecke liked to call him — yes, he'd been knighted by the Queen in 2006 — was probably the world's foremost epidemiologist.

He had published more than 450 scientific articles, and was one of two authors behind *Infectious Diseases of Humans: dynamics and control* — the most cited book in the field. He had served as an adviser to the Bill and Melinda Gates Foundation.

Giesecke wasn't a fan of his. After all, Anderson had been in charge of the group producing those models — the ones that had sparked so many overreactions.

On top of that, Anderson, in his previous role as advisor to the British government, had been part of raising the swine flu to a level six in the UK — before the WHO.

When the WHO followed suit and declared that the world had been struck by a pandemic, those contracts binding several of the world's countries to buy vaccines from drug companies were activated. One such contract had provided Sweden and Anders Tegnell with 18 million doses of Pandemrix from GlaxoSmithKline.

But it was as though no dirt ever stuck to the British patriarch.

'Sir Roy is very arrogant, too. Ferguson takes after his dad.'

If Giesecke held certain opinions about Ferguson's personality, his university, and his intellectual mentor, it was still nothing compared to Giesecke's thoughts about Ferguson's scientific models.

In his eyes, Ferguson's career was one long string of disastrous miscalculations with fateful consequences. The problem, Giesecke argued, was that epidemiological forecasts were often about people. These weren't like Einstein's models about light bending around a celestial body. They weren't like Newton's laws of motion. This was a social science.

And yet the world's journalists and decision-makers seemed to put a great deal of faith in mathematical models.

This was nothing new. It was the same with economic forecasts. They never turned out to be true either. Weren't there statistics on how bad economists were at predicting recessions? Yet everyone listened to them.

'Fortune tellers and magicians. They've always had a high standing in any society.'

It made it even worse that the report in mid-March came from the UK of all places — and that it led the country to switch its strategy. Sure, the

British were a bit supercilious, but London was still a bit like the Rome of epidemiology. That's where Nobel Prize winners came from; that's where you went if you were someone.

Giesecke himself had worked there a long time before. One of his favourite anecdotes was about how he wasn't allowed to give blood in Sweden because he'd lived in England for more than a year while mad cow disease was raging.

Anders Tegnell and the Public Health Agency had been leaning heavily on the British government's line. As recently as the day before the Imperial report came out, Tegnell had told *Aftonbladet* that they were the 'best in the world', and that 'heavy British research' showed the Swedish strategy was correct.

Up until now, Sweden had only had one ally in its view of the virus. But because it was the UK, it had been all right. So the Brits making a U-turn was bad for Sweden.

In truth, Johan Giesecke was too old. But now he was about to take on the UK's newly appointed chief magician.

Attempting the impossible

On the surface, perhaps it all looked like a mere accident. Someone in China had worked up an appetite for some boiled bat — or perhaps a little deep-fried pangolin. Who knew? A new virus had spread across the world, making a few highly educated noblemen and academics, with all their good intentions, wrangle over the right way forward. That wasn't so strange, was it?

But behind the conflict now brewing between the world's epidemiologists, there was a bigger, almost philosophical, question: was it even possible to use complex modelling to foresee how an infection would spread through society?

It all began in the US in 2001. Just a week after the terrorist attacks on September 11, letters containing anthrax spores began to appear in politicians' mailboxes and newspaper offices. Five people died, and another 17 were infected. The investigation that followed would become one of the biggest in the history of the FBI.

The military and healthcare experts began to worry about a wave of bioterrorism. There were plenty of viruses, spores, and bacteria to release. The worst pathogen of them all — the smallpox virus — may have been eradicated, but it still existed in at least two laboratories in the US and Russia. Ever since the last known case, in Somalia in 1977, there had been a debate about whether these virus samples should be destroyed. Some experts argued there was a risk the samples could end up in the wrong hands, while others claimed there was great scientific value in keeping them. After all, no one could be certain the two known samples were the only ones in existence.

In the autumn of 2001, the US National Institutes of Health called several meetings about the new threat. The agency was the biggest research funder in the world, and now it wanted to find out whether it was possible to use mathematical modelling to strengthen protection against bioterrorism.

It had been three centuries since John Graunt and Daniel Bernoulli lived and worked. It had been roughly a hundred years since Ross, Topley, Hedrich, and the others.

Indeed, a few things had happened. When the world's doctors vaccinated children against measles and mumps, health agencies could calculate how many jabs were needed for herd immunity to kick in and the population to be protected. When salmonella spread through a city, epidemiologists could use statistical methods to find the source. If a new drug was approved, it was possible to calculate the probability of side effects. And it was all done with the help of Fisher's exact test, the null hypothesis, and other statistical advances.

But compared to other disciplines, the use of scientific modelling remained limited. The epidemiological literature may not have been easy reading, but most of the maths wasn't more advanced than what a gifted upper-secondary school student could have grasped.

Epidemiology hadn't developed in the same direction as chemistry or physics, where mathematical modelling combined with increasingly powerful computers had taken existing knowledge further and further into the stratosphere, more and more incomprehensible to lay people.

An epidemiologist couldn't simply model the spread of an infection in a computer the same way an engineer could model the aerodynamic resistance of an aeroplane wing.

Not yet, anyway.

The first meeting at the National Institutes of Health took place in December 2001. Among the invited guests were health experts, epidemiologists, and experts in scientific modelling.

Just a few months earlier, the United Kingdom had been affected by an outbreak of foot-and-mouth disease. The models used on this occasion appeared to have worked to forecast the spread of the virus.

Together, the scientists at the meeting in the US arrived at the conclusion that epidemiological models could be of great value. Not to forecast how many would die if al-Qaeda planted smallpox virus in 10 US airports, but to compare different scenarios — and thus establish which political and medical interventions would be most effective.

Two years later, Neil Ferguson published an article in the journal *Nature* titled 'Planning for Smallpox Outbreaks'. His conclusions were rather humble. Using models to identify an optimal strategy was 'attempting the impossible', he wrote.

But at least it was a start.

Johan Giesecke, too, was lured into the magic business. Around the same time as the Brits and the Americans began to apply their models, he started up a group called 'S-GEM', or the Stockholm Group for Epidemic Modeling. It was an interdisciplinary network of doctors, sociologists, mathematicians, statisticians, programmers, and other researchers. Together, they would develop methods for applying models to study the effects of vaccination programmes, the transmission of infectious diseases in sexual networks, the development of resistant bacteria, and other things that interested infectious-disease doctors.

One project, started in 2004, was known as MicroSim. It was a model based on public information about all the nine million people living in Sweden at the time.

Its features were virtually Orwellian. Every Swede was coded, using their personal identity number, place of residence, the location of their workplace or school, their parents' personal-identity numbers, their family type, age, sex, and other things. The country's surface was divided into tiny squares.

Its specificity made it unique. Nowhere in the world was there a model this detailed.

But, over the years, Johan Giesecke had become increasingly sceptical of overly complex epidemic models.

The results could end up being wrong. Very wrong. There were so many parameters involved, and changing the value of just one of them was enough to make the entire output look completely different.

For behind every parameter lay an assumption. If, for example, you assumed that closing schools would radically reduce transmission — well, then, the end result would also show that shutting down schools was effective. Despite this, the models seemed confidence-inspiring and impressive. All those Greek letters and integrals and whatnot made them look more credible than they actually were.

That was the big danger. They could create a false sense of security. It wasn't possible to escape the fact that, in the end, all models were based on an estimation of what the real world was like.

With every inaccurate forecast broadcast from London, Giesecke's scepticism of models was reinforced. Events showed it was better to be moderately talented in mathematics.

Johan Giesecke was moderately talented.

Anders Tegnell was moderately talented, too, he thought.

So while the rest of the world went on a journey into the world of mathematics, Giesecke stayed put in the epidemiology of the early 2000s.

For 11 years, it had been a strictly academic debate. Many of the big epidemics since 2009 — such as cholera in Haiti in 2010, MERS in the Middle East in 2012, or the 2019 measles outbreak in New Zealand — had been limited to a certain part of the world.

This time, it was different: this was a global pandemic. The conflict between the maths nerds and the maths sceptics — lying dormant since 2001 — was suddenly flaring up.

And now the first group was receiving help from a *Star Wars*–loving entrepreneur from California.

The hammer and the dance

On the same day that the report from Imperial College was released, a 37-year-old Spaniard was putting the finishing touches to what would become one of the most read texts of the year.

Tomas Pueyo loved stories. His father was a filmmaker, and throughout his childhood the two of them had talked about everything from Shakespeare plays to Hollywood productions.

It was human to love them, he liked to say. It was evolutionarily determined. Those who loved stories could memorise more information and solve more problems, thus surviving to a greater extent. They, in turn, would have children who also carried the story-loving gene.

Despite his interest in books and films, Tomas Pueyo chose to train as an engineer — first in Madrid and then in Paris. Eventually, he set off to the US for an MBA at Stanford.

His career was fairly typical of the international elite emerging in the decades that followed the new millennium. He spent a few years in the consulting industry, and another few at some global companies, before getting stuck in the Silicon Valley startup world. There, he started out working for two companies making Facebook games, then at an investment platform, before ending up in a high-ranking position at a company working with digital teaching solutions. The company's name was Course Hero, and it was one of Silicon Valley's many 'unicorns' — an epithet given to a newly founded company valued at more than $1 billion.

His interest in storytelling made him stand out a bit. Two years earlier, he'd written the book *The Star Wars Rings: the hidden structure behind the Star Wars story*, describing the film series' dramatic arc and attempting to decipher some of the riddles in the story. In his mild, precise voice, he also gave talks on the subject. One of his presentations had been published on the TED platform, but so far not many had seen it.

Once reports about the new virus began to trickle in, first from China, and then from northern Italy, Tomas Pueyo recognised what he saw.

This was exponential growth.

Exponential growth is a phenomenon explaining the way much of the world works. If something — a virus, a bacterium, GDP, wealth, the number of transistors that can fit onto a chip — increases by 5, 10, or 20 per cent per day or year, and continues to do so, something almost magical happens.

If, for example, an app has 10,000 users and grows by 20 per cent each month, a month later it will have 12,000 users. That might not seem like a big difference.

It won't look particularly impressive the next month either, when the user base has grown to 14,400. But a year later, the number of users will be almost 130,000 — and the year after that, users will number one million. Yet another year later, the corresponding figure will be 10 million. The following year? Ninety-one million.

The same phenomenon is sometimes called 'compound interest'. Finance people like to attribute a quote referring to exponential growth as the eighth wonder of the world to Albert Einstein: 'He who understands it earns it … he who doesn't pays it.'

Einstein probably never said that, but the fact that many people have a hard time grasping the power of accumulated capital is beyond doubt.

The apocryphal story about the man who invented chess is both a tale about the phenomenon itself and about the difficulty in understanding it. Most people have heard it before. The inventor of chess asks his ruler for one grain of rice for the first square on the board, two grains for the second, four for the next, and so on. The ruler in the story agrees to his proposition, without realising that the final amount ends up being thousands of times more than the entire world's rice production.

Tomas Pueyo understood exponential growth. It was impossible to work in Silicon Valley without doing so. The entire digital economy was held up by this magic.

Pueyo started studying the epidemiological literature. He searched online for studies and scientific reports on how the coronavirus behaved. There was plenty of information. For a few years now, scientists had been able to post finished but unreviewed manuscripts to online repositories such as medRxiv and bioRxiv. The names of these repositories were pronounced 'med-archive' and 'bio-archive' in a little game of wordplay for the initiated: as a common statistical method called the 'x^2 test' was also known as the 'chi-squared test', the x could be exchanged for the letters 'chi'. Among the financial backers of these websites were the Facebook founder Mark Zuckerberg's organisation the Chan Zuckerberg Initiative.

Over the course of the Covid spring, these repositories would see many new visitors. Laypeople across the world attempted to interpret, analyse, and forecast the spread of the virus.

Tomas Pueyo was one of them. But unlike many others, he had both a scientific background and an ability to express himself.

What's more, he had a platform. He sat down and started writing a text for a site called Medium.

Like medRxiv and bioRxiv, Medium was another novelty with roots in Silicon Valley. It had been founded in 2012 by Evan Williams, who had also been part of launching Twitter. Over the years, it had grown into a much-read hybrid between professional journalism and a blogging platform. Several reputable papers — including *The New York Times*, *The Atlantic*, and *The New Yorker* — posted texts to Medium, but anyone could create an account and start typing. In February 2019, the Amazon founder Jeff Bezos had published a text where he revealed that *The National Enquirer* knew of his romantic affair and had tried to blackmail him.

Like much else created in Silicon Valley, Medium was a tool for disrupting power structures within journalism, science, and economics.

The first text by Tomas Pueyo was published on 10 March with the title 'Coronavirus: why you must act now'. It described how the virus was spreading outside China. His message was that its increase was exponential, and the number of cases was greater than many thought.

In one of his charts, he drew a line corresponding to a daily growth rate of 40 per cent. In countries with a rate higher than that, the number of cases was doubling every other day. Sweden ended up on the wrong side of the line — a little better than Malaysia and Australia, and a little worse than Greece.

The text was picked up in Stockholm, too. Denis Coulombier read it, and was impressed by the graphical representation. He sent it to Johan von Schreeb and Jan Albert.

'A highly convincing message. Time to shut down schools and gatherings in Stockholm.'

Jan Albert forwarded the text to a few people at the Public Health Agency, among them Anders Tegnell: 'I don't have enough knowledge of pros and cons to have an opinion. I trust your judgement.'

Tegnell read Pueyo's text and replied: 'The facts seem very soft.'

But around the world, millions of people were reading his analysis with eyes a lot less critical — as well as Pueyo's recipe for how the world's politicians should act.

Just like the Swedes, Pueyo wanted to 'flatten the curve' — that is, to delay the course of the epidemic as much as possible. But for Pueyo, the way to do that involved 'keeping people home as much as possible, for as long as possible'. Statistics from China showed that it could be done. Statistics from the Spanish flu showed it, too — Pueyo had found the story about Philadelphia and St Louis as well.

Based on figures from Hubei Province, Pueyo interpreted the risk of dying if infected with the coronavirus as somewhere between 3.8 and 4 per cent. This meant that the fatality rate was twice as high as that of the Spanish flu — and 30 times higher than a regular seasonal influenza.

But it wasn't quite that simple. Its deadliness depended on multiple factors, not least of which was the age distribution in each country.

The most important thing was that the healthcare system didn't collapse. Countries that were prepared and acted quickly, he wrote, could reduce the death toll by a factor of ten.

But what should countries that had not yet been hit do?

On 17 March — the day after the report from Imperial College became known — Tomas Pueyo offered his answer to that question. The text he posted was titled 'The Hammer and the Dance'.

His message was that the governments of the world should act swiftly and forcefully — bringing down the hammer — to get the spread of the virus under control. This would give societies time to buttress their healthcare systems, build up their testing capacity, and — most of all — learn more. He included a graph showing the number of scientific articles published about the virus since January. By now, the number of studies on PubMed, ChemRxiv, arXiv, medRxiv, and bioRxiv had gone from zero at the start of the year to almost 300. Perhaps a vaccine wasn't far away.

His view on adopting a herd-immunity approach was clear. It would mean 10 million deaths in the US alone — 25 times more than the Americans who perished in the Second World War.

He extended his military metaphor: 'The US (and presumably the UK) are about to go to war without armor,' he wrote.

He'd arrived at his figure of 10 million by using a data model posted to GitHub — a web-hosting service for storing open-source code.

The model allowed you to set your own R_0 number, mortality rate, and other things. Pueyo entered an R_0 of 2.4, and set the percentage of infected individuals who'd end up in hospital at 14. He set the case fatality rate at 4 per cent. But disaster could be avoided. If the world's governments applied the hammer first, they could then initiate what he called the 'dance of R'. By introducing a number of measures to reduce transmission, they could balance the R number, keeping it below or close to 1. While waiting for a vaccine, the epidemic could thus be kept in check.

The hammer and the dance: with his poetic description, Tomas Pueyo managed to distil decades of epidemiological literature. The expression went viral — in the newer, digital sense of the word. More than 40 million people read his text, and Pueyo, who hadn't known the first thing about epidemiology just a week before, was contacted by and invited to advise politicians and other decision-makers from the US, Latin America, and Europe.

His message was the same as in the text. And thanks to a tool on Medium, it would later be possible to see what section of the text had been highlighted the most by readers: 'Countries can fight,' it read. 'They can lock down for a few weeks to buy us time, create an educated action plan, and control this virus until we have a vaccine.'

Pueyo's story spread across the world.

The model that wasn't used

Johan Giesecke settled in quickly at his old agency. No one seemed to find it strange that he — the state epidemiologist from two generations ago — was now waltzing around the corridors.

In his time, they'd all had their own offices, but now the agency had implemented 'activity-based' workstations. It meant Giesecke always had to walk around looking for the people he wanted to talk to. On top of that, he suffered from what he liked to call an inverted form of *l'esprit de l'escalier*.

The meaning of the expression is something like 'staircase wit', and it usually means coming up with an intelligent rejoinder several minutes too late. For Giesecke, it worked a little differently. He would realise that someone had said something clever several hours after they'd said it. Sometimes days later. So he ended up wandering around the corridors quite a bit, seeking out a person who'd had an interesting theory a few days before.

Giesecke worked relatively short days. He tried to show up in time for the morning meeting with the heads of the different units, and then he replied to emails, talked to people, and read scientific articles until lunch. Which he usually had with Anders Tegnell.

At 1.00 pm, it was time for the epidemic situation meeting. There, he took up quite a bit of space. Mostly he complained about poorly executed charts.

At 4.00 pm, he would gather up his papers, tuck his snus can into his pocket, and drive back home to Södertälje.

At the time, the plan was still for the agency to use MicroSim to produce a model of the spread of the new coronavirus. To Sweden's Radio, whose science desk kept a close eye on the agency's modelling efforts, Lisa Brouwers said it would happen soon. The analysis unit was just waiting for slightly better data. It was, for instance, not yet entirely clear how many of the infected were asymptomatic. It also wasn't clear how many people already carried the virus.

But the model had led them astray once before. It was a calculation using MicroSim that had generated the positive results in support of a mass vaccination of the Swedish population in 2009. It had showed that administering Pandemrix to all Swedes to be 'very cost effective'.

Johan Giesecke aired his scepticism. He wasn't particularly fond of the idea of using such an advanced transmission model to predict how the new virus would move through society. Even this early, it was possible to study the results generated by other advanced models.

Two months prior — on 31 January — *The Lancet* had published a forecast of the spread of the virus, nationally and internationally. Among other things, it had analysed air traffic between Wuhan and the rest of the world — and had arrived at the conclusion that Sydney, in Australia, had received the most travellers from there. This had led a few well-versed doctors and epidemiologists to warn against travelling there.

But, for some inexplicable reason, northern Italy had been struck the hardest.

At the Swedish Public Health Agency, the model-sceptical stance slowly began to gain ground.

MicroSim ended up staying in the drawer.

A puzzle

On the evening of 17 March, Johan von Schreeb sent a copy of the Imperial report to eight people at the Karolinska Institute. Among the recipients were Jan Albert and Johan Giesecke, who was a professor emeritus at the university and thus retained an email address connected to it.

'Hi. Key report now making the UK change its strategy from mitigation to suppression,' he wrote.

The word 'mitigation' was a term for the strategy chosen by the Public Health Agency. Its focus was to dampen the effects of the virus — not to prevent transmission at all costs.

'Suppression', on the other hand, meant attempting to stamp out the virus as much as possible.

Now, pressure on the Public Health Agency would be high, von Schreeb predicted.

'Read and have a think,' he wrote.

Within public-health policy, the opposition between the two strategies had become a never-ending saga. And it didn't just apply to infectious-disease epidemiology. For decades, drug policy had been dominated by these two competing approaches. There were those who believed that drug use was an unavoidable consequence of what the world looked like, and thus thought policy should focus on alleviating the negative consequences of substance abuse. And there were those who believed that drug use should be avoided at all costs.

Within drug-policy debates, these two strategies were known as harm reduction and zero tolerance. For instance, those who advocated harm reduction wanted to offer clean needles and substitution therapy to heroin addicts, and to decriminalise drug use in order to make it easier for people to seek treatment.

Conversely, those who wanted zero tolerance called for harsher penalties, and thought all treatment should be focused on achieving complete freedom from drugs.

The Swedish stance had long been zero tolerance. Starting in the 1960s, pretty well all Swedish politicians had looked at drug use from an epidemiological perspective. Narcomania was thought of as a socially communicable state.

As international research increasingly began to advocate harm-reduction measures, the Swedish line had softened. But the Public Health Agency wanted to go further than Swedish politicians and, for instance, look into decriminalising private use.

Clamp down hard? Or dampen the consequences? This was the philosophical and ethical dilemma permeating everything from infectious-disease control to sexual-health policy. Was it better to encourage young people to practise sexual abstinence, or to distribute condoms at upper-secondary schools? Was it preferrable to increase penalties for drunk driving, or subsidise night taxis?

Now, in March 2020, country after country were choosing hardline policies.

They declared war on the virus.

Would Sweden follow suit?

Jan Albert read the Imperial report. Then he called Tom Britton.

Albert and Britton had known each other for a few years. They had conducted HIV research together and had published a few articles on the transmission of that virus. Now, Albert wanted to hear Britton's take on the British figures.

Tom Britton knew Neil Ferguson a little. They had met at a conference on the Isle of Skye, off the west coast of Scotland, in the late 1990s.

Britton had a habit of saving group photos from every conference he'd been to. From the walls of his study, hundreds of mathematicians and epidemiologists gazed down at him as he worked.

In one of the faded photographs, just above eye height, hung the image of a smiling Neil Ferguson. He'd dressed differently back then. In his red cardigan, he looked more like a caricature of a British lord — like the human member of the *Wallace and Gromit* duo — than the professor in urban clothing he'd now become.

Britton remembered Ferguson as a pleasant and smart guy. Well spoken like a British politician; sharp like a Japanese knife.

Britton skimmed the report, and immediately found a few things he thought were strange. But he didn't make much of them at the time. There was a bigger problem.

The suppression scenario laid out in the report was completely unrealistic. Why would you paralyse all of society — thus sparking mass unemployment, uprisings, and sudden poverty — for a disease with such a low fatality rate?

It would never work.

Jan Albert agreed. It was unreasonable to propose such pervasive measures without also calculating the harmful effects on society, the collateral damage.

The way Jan Albert saw it, the task was to identify the optimal level of restrictions. Buying time for a limited period was sensible, but if a lot of companies, businesses, and restaurants went under, it could lead to economic effects and a reduced tax base that, in turn, would mean less money for the healthcare system.

It was a puzzle that had to be solved, he thought.

But should it really be up to some doctors at the Karolinska Institute and the Public Health Agency to solve it? Wasn't this a job for the country's politicians?

On the same day — 17 March — the government called a closed-door meeting with the leaders of all the parties represented in the Swedish parliament. Prime Minister Stefan Löfven now explained the strategy that was not yet official but would eventually be published on the government's website three weeks later.

There were six different parts to the strategy: reducing the rate of transmission; ensuring sufficient resources to the healthcare system; limiting harmful effects on other activities essential to society; alleviating consequences for citizens and companies; allaying fear in society; and introducing the right measures at the right time.

'The measures taken by the government in the past and moving forward are based on the expertise and knowledge of the authorities. And on their recommendations,' he said.

Also participating in the meeting was Johan Carlson. The baseline of the strategy, he said, was to separate the healthy from the sick.

This may have sounded self-evident, but as the Imperial report now spread around the world, governments would soon be applying a very different strategy.

They would start locking up healthy people.

About this, however, the participants in the meeting were still unaware. Instead, a discussion ensued as to whether it was really the Public Health Agency that should be deciding all these issues.

The background was that Anders Tegnell, in an interview with the evening newspaper *Expressen* a few days previously, had been asked whether the whole country should do as the company Spotify had done, which was to tell all its employees to work from home.

In the interview, Tegnell reasoned that only certain groups in society had the means to do so, and the question thus came with an equity dimension. Nevertheless, the day before the meeting with the party leaders — 16 March — Tegnell had recommended that all Stockholmers who could work from home should do so.

It did indeed appear as though the Public Health Agency had begun to make the types of decisions that politicians were paid to make. Perhaps they were engaged in a puzzle that another occupational group should be solving?

When Löfven yielded the floor on 17 March, he said it was important that the government followed the agency's advice. He didn't seem to think that Tegnell was stepping into the domain of politics: 'Pointing to the trade-offs that have to be made is good, I think. To be able to make the best decision possible.'

Calculating in the dark

The eighteenth of March was a Wednesday. The world's leaders continued to bring down Tomas Pueyo's metaphorical hammer. Belgium imposed a lockdown. The longest land border in the world — between the US and Canada — was closed to non-essential travel.

But in Sweden, a group of scientists continued to dissect the Imperial report.

Early in the morning, Jan Albert replied to von Schreeb's email.

'My sense is that this virus is too fast-footed to let itself be affected by "sensible" measures. Is it better to pull the bad tooth quickly or slowly? Stowing away the elderly is probably good, though.'

He added both Anders Tegnell and Tom Britton to the email thread. Now there was a whole band of them.

Johan Giesecke was the one who had got the farthest. Just on page four, he'd found several dubious assumptions by Ferguson.

Giesecke jotted down his initial thoughts in an email.

'I think the most serious issue is that the authors estimate transmission to happen 1/3 within the family, 1/3 in schools or at work, and 1/3 out in society.'

This didn't correspond to the data produced by the WHO, among others. A delegation from the organisation that had been to China estimated transmission within the family to account for 80 per cent.

'Even here, the report's analysis of the spread is way off the mark,' Giesecke wrote.

He also seized on the opportunity to account for Ferguson's merits and epidemiological pedigree — updating everyone on the family feud, so to speak: 'Remember, when Roy Anderson's group (now led by Neil Ferguson) projected the death toll for mad cow disease 25 years ago, they set the upper limit at 200,000.'

The email thread grew. Step by step, the Swedes picked apart the British figures.

Tom Britton noted that Ferguson assumed only 50 per cent would comply with quarantine recommendations. That might be true of the UK, but his guess was that Swedes were a little more obedient and risk-aware.

Johan Giesecke found more problems. Ferguson had assumed the hospital capacity would remain unchanged. But even now, the world's countries were rapidly expanding their intensive-care capacity.

After lunch, the state epidemiologist added his first contribution: 'Just a thought, I don't know if my reasoning is correct,' he began. 'There seems to be an assumption of a fairly low number of unknown cases, which should lead to underestimating the rate of transmission and heavily overestimating the proportion that gets sick. Hence the extremely pessimistic forecasts and the notion of how difficult it'll be to reach herd immunity.'

Two days later — Friday 20 March — Tom Britton had finished perusing the study. Early in the morning, he sent his thoughts to the group.

'Two assumptions are that circa 50 per cent of all cases in China were reported, and another is that the deadliness is 0.9 per cent.'

It wasn't entirely clear in the report, Britton thought, but his interpretation was that the fatality figure had been based on an estimate of the total number of infections — not on reported cases.

This was an important distinction. If the death toll was expressed in proportion to the number of reported cases, and if those only amounted to half of all infections, it would mean that the actual fatality ate was only half as high: 0.45 per cent.

Regardless, Britton didn't think the numbers sounded right. He'd seen other assessments pointing to a fatality rate significantly lower than 0.9 per cent.

Either the Chinese death toll was wrong, or the proportion of discovered cases was low. Either way, it would translate into a lower fatality rate.

'Both of these would be positive changes — that is, indicate fewer deaths in Sweden,' Britton wrote.

He wanted to study this closer, but couldn't find any good studies to use.

'Could anyone help with this?'

Finding out how many had been infected was crucial. Without that piece of the puzzle, no one could calculate with any certainty how dangerous the virus was. The mortality measure was known as IFR — infection fatality rate — and was calculated by a simple division: the number of deaths divided by the number of infections.

A few weeks earlier, the WHO had managed to strike fear into the world by reporting a case fatality rate of 3.4 per cent. But that number was just as meaningless as it was terrifying. At that time, those who had been tested were people with severe symptoms, thus ending up in hospital. The risk of those individuals dying was significantly higher than for the average, not-yet-infected person out in society.

The actual fatality rate was surely lower than 3 per cent. But how much lower?

A few minutes later, Anders Tegnell replied. He couldn't help Britton with scientific references, but his impression was that far fewer than half of all cases had been identified in China.

'As soon as there is more widespread testing, they're finding large numbers of people without symptoms.'

He therefore guessed that the number of hidden cases was large — probably 10 or 20 times what had been reported.

But no one knew for sure.

It was not an easy situation. Now, the Swedish group had a division with an uncertain denominator. And in possession of the coveted figure was a shady regime in faraway Asia.

They were calculating in the dark.

Anders Tegnell wondered why the Chinese were playing this game. It had been more than two and a half months since the first case was discovered in Wuhan. By this time, the Chinese should have had a lot more information than they were letting the world in on. How many had really been infected?

This, he wrote to the group, was 'one of the mysteries now'.

Could any of the researchers at the Karolinska Institute help him?

The Karolinska Institute was the pride of the nation. It was the only seat of learning in Sweden — in all of the Nordic countries — that placed high in the rankings of prestigious universities regularly compiled by innumerable media outlets and other organisations.

It had been founded in 1810 with the aim of producing barber surgeons for the Swedish military power that had lost half the country to the Russians the year before. But over time, the university became a magnet for scientists from all over the world. Since 1901, the institute had also selected the annual recipient of the Nobel Prize in medicine.

Among those who had been copied in on the thread was one of the Karolinska Institute's workhorses. His name was Matti Sällberg, and he led a group of researchers already working on a vaccine against the new virus.

Sällberg had a bit of a peculiar background. He was a biomedical analyst, but had also completed an entire degree in dentistry alongside his doctorate.

Ever since January, Sällberg had applied his full mental bandwidth to SARS-CoV-2. He'd put all other work aside and locked himself in his closet-like room, reading everything he could find about the new virus. If there were any in the world who knew more about SARS-CoV-2 by mid-March, there probably weren't many of them.

In the last few weeks, Sällberg had thus become a bit of a celebrity. He appeared on television and in the big newspapers. Journalists came to visit him in his little closet, and took his photo from every angle.

He hadn't actually worn a white lab coat in a long time — mostly he sat in front of the computer. Besides, he preferred stylish sportcoats with a little handkerchief tucked into the breast pocket. But now, there were so many photographers — and they wanted him in full uniform. So he rose to the occasion, pulling on his coat and gazing into the camera with steely-grey eyes.

Sällberg made a brief appearance in the email thread. He agreed with Anders Tegnell that it was peculiar that no long-term follow-ups were being done. At the same time, there was clearly a large proportion of unknown cases. In other words, the number of infections was a lot higher than many thought — and the mortality rate was lower.

'Herd immunity is what will get this under control,' he wrote.

Then one of Sällberg's colleagues jumped into the discussion. His name was Anders Sönnerborg, and he was a professor of infectious diseases. He had several contacts in China, and had asked them about the mystery.

'I've put the question to my Chinese contacts but [have] not received an answer. I'll chase them on it.'

They'd have to continue guessing about the true deadliness of the new virus. The mystery would have to wait for its solution.

'You can't help but wonder what's going on here,' Tegnell concluded.

The china shop

It wasn't just in Stockholm that people were sinking their teeth into the report from London.

In Umeå, the professor Joacim Rocklöv and seven other scientists began to create a Swedish scenario based on the Imperial report. After just a few days, they published their unreviewed study online. It showed that the need for intensive-care beds would exceed the Swedish capacity many times over.

In the most likely scenario, there would be a need for 1,600 to 8,300 beds at most — but perhaps as many as 14,000. The need would thus be between four and 20 times greater than Sweden's capacity.

Their report gained a lot of attention. Right away, Sweden's Television did a news story and interviewed Rocklöv. 'What we're seeing is that it's important to do a lot, and more. We can work remotely and close schools to the extent that's possible. We can find lots of different measures,' he said.

The press officer at the Public Health Agency told Sweden's Television that they didn't wish to comment on the figures from Umeå, but Anders Tegnell still read the report. He thought it contained several errors, called it a 'horror scenario of no use to anyone', and wrote to Johan von Schreeb, Tom Britton, Johan Giesecke, and several others, telling them that it was probably 'straight-up plagiarised from Imperial's latest report'.

He asked Johan Giesecke to read it carefully and comment on it in the media.

In a statement to Sweden's Television, Giesecke said: 'The model assumes that everyone mixes together, which isn't true in Sweden.'

At the same time, a similar project was initiated at Uppsala University. Lynn Kamerlin, Peter Kasson, and four other researchers borrowed supercomputers in four different cities to crunch the numbers on a model of their own. Quite similar to MicroSim, it contained detailed information about the age, occupations, and geographical locations of the Swedish population, which was complemented by cultural parameters borrowed from studies of other countries.

When the calculation was ready, it would show that 96,000 Swedes could perish by 1 July — if the strategy wasn't changed.

With the Imperial report — and the version from Umeå — the spotlight once again turned to the Government Offices. For the past couple of weeks, officials and politicians had been saying to journalists that they had chosen the scientific route. They had listened to their expert agency. Unlike the rest of the world, they hadn't been lured into closing down society in a show of decisiveness, they said proudly.

Many seasoned political reporters were surprised by their choice of words. Never before had Swedish decision-makers so clearly painted a conflict between science and politics.

For things were rarely that simple. A professor of economics and a professor of environmental science both dealt in science, but could still have diametrically opposed opinions about the propriety of opening a nickel mine in Lapland. What did the *science* say about the continuing shutdown of Swedish nuclear power plants?

One of the government's tasks was to weigh different viewpoints against each other. This, too, they appeared to have delegated to the Public Health Agency.

And it was enough to read any news article written outside Stockholm to realise that there were plenty of scientists who saw the pandemic from an entirely different perspective. It wasn't just panic-stricken Italian and French people who advocated a lockdown. There were British epidemiologists, German micro-biologists, professors in Umeå.

The government could no longer put off the problem. There was no single scientific path. There were only two options: follow the Public Health Agency's strategy — and sit back; or do like other countries — and close down society.

The Swedish constitution offered no protection. The government may not have been able to govern the agency, but there was nothing stopping it from ignoring the agency's assessments and introducing more extensive restrictions of its own. It was possible for the government to take over. The governments of Denmark and Norway had already made decisions that went against the advice of their agencies.

And it was possible to go even further. In Germany, chancellor Angela Merkel — who did, admittedly, hold a doctor's degree in quantum chemistry — went on TV to explain how R numbers worked.

The problem with the second option — taking charge — was that everyone who knew anything about infectious-disease control, epidemiology, or scientific modelling worked at the Public Health Agency — not the Government Offices. That's how the Swedish system was structured. Unlike in many other countries, the government had no chief medical officer able to make their own assessments. There was no scientific adviser who could evaluate the agency's conclusions. Compared to other countries, the Swedish Government Offices were small next to its government agencies. Who were *they* — a group of lawyers and political scientists, some crisis-management expert hastily called in from the Swedish Defence University, under the leadership of the prime minister, an old union rep from somewhere up north — to override some two dozen epidemiologists who seemed to be in terrifying agreement?

And then cook up a new strategy in a week's time? No, no, no.

'It would be like marching into a china shop,' said one of the people involved.

The china shop was the Public Health Agency's strategy: a complex set of interventions and measures based on generations of knowledge.

There was no way the Government Offices could purchase new china. Not on such short notice. They'd simply end up gluing together broken pieces for the rest of the year. What's more, both officials and politicians felt they would have to own the Swedish strategy for all eternity should they choose to change it. No one was thrilled about that.

There was also a significant consensus that the strategy was reasonable. Sure, the Public Health Agency may have got off to a slow start. But the extensive lockdowns in Europe felt panicked.

Besides, every public opinion survey indicated that the people supported the strategy. The agency enjoyed a high level of confidence. Even the confidence in the government began to tick upward.

Sweden remained open.

The pension fund manager

Kerstin Hessius strode around her apartment on Östermalm in Stockholm. She had a bit of a stuffy nose, was working from home, and was considering whether to cancel her participation in a panel due to take place two days later.

It wasn't just the cold that made her hesitate. The whole arrangement felt a little off. As the program had long been decided, she was supposed to speak on sustainability issues. But she didn't really feel like harping on about palm oil plantations, fossil-fuel divestments, and miners' rights when the world economy was being sucked into a black hole. In a month, the value of the shares on the Stockholm stock exchange had fallen by 30 per cent.

So she called up the organisers and explained that she was sick.

'What a shame,' the man on the other end of the line replied. 'I'd planned to move you to another seminar.'

He explained the new concept: Hessius and two other economists would have been speaking about the economic effects of the Covid-19 pandemic.

Damn it, she thought.

Now she wanted to join again. But she was too well-mannered to change her mind twice in one minute. So she hung up, and continued to watch the devastation from her apartment.

Kerstin Hessius was 61 years old, with a long career behind her. Some 21 years earlier, she had been pronounced the most powerful woman in Swedish business. Since then she may have been surpassed by a younger talent or two, but there was no question as to whether she remained powerful. If anyone was planning a communist revolution and wanted a list of ideological enemies, they could have laminated and saved the list of members in Hessius's network that had once been published in the business magazine *Veckans Affärer*: it included top executives, business tycoons, union reps, media bosses, and politicians.

Her Stockholm dialect still flowed as rapidly as before, peppered with a few curses — nothing crude, just a couple of adverbs swapped out here and there as required for emphasis. After all, she hailed from the Stockholm stockmarket floor, not New York's.

She'd also been handed quite a bit of money to manage. It wasn't her own, but then again that's rarely the case in this world. As the CEO of the Third Swedish National Pension Fund, Kerstin Hessius was in charge of more than 400 billion SEK in Swedish pension savings.

Though now it was considerably less.

The national pension funds served as a buffer in the Swedish pension system. In the years when pension contributions outstripped payouts, the surplus was put into one of the funds — imaginatively named by numbers: first, second, third, and so on.

In the years when the payouts were higher — as they tended to be these days, with an increasingly ageing population — the funds pitched in some additional money.

With each passing day, her fund was decreasing in value.

Where would it end?

The finance industry is a future machine. Risks and possibilities are weighed, analysed, priced, and sent back and forth across the world. Kerstin Hessius had worked inside the machine her entire life. She'd held jobs at funds, at banks, and as the deputy governor of Riksbanken, Sweden's central bank.

Now, she remembered 11 September 2001. How they'd heard about the first plane crashing into the World Trade Center, turned on their bulky TVs, then watched the second plane fly in.

She'd been CEO of the Stockholm stock exchange back then. And for the first time, she understood what the term 'financial instability' truly meant.

No one could put a price on risk. The market vanished. The machine stopped, and the future went, too.

That time, the uncertainty lasted a short period. Only a few days. This crisis — the Covid crisis — had already lasted longer. And still people only talked about the virus, about the death toll, about lockdowns, about even more lockdowns. No one wanted — or dared — to talk about the time after. This wasn't so much a Covid crisis as a lockdown crisis.

She thought of early autumn 2008. After Lehman Brothers had gone bankrupt, it was as though decision-makers didn't see, or didn't want to see, what was about to happen. The politicians were slow; so was the Riksbank.

On 8 October 2008, she wrote an op-ed taking aim at the Swedish Riksbank. She wanted it to stop focusing solely on the inflation target.

'Hello, dear old colleagues,' she wrote, 'it's time to wake up and live in the present.'

Perhaps she ought to do something similar now?

She decided she was feeling well enough.

The next day, Thursday 19 March, she sat on that panel, feeling herself getting properly worked up. All the other two economists wanted to talk about were financial details. Hessius wanted to discuss whether lockdowns were the way to go at all. Was it right to close down all of society to stop the spread of the virus?

What did they want to achieve? What was the objective of policies in countries declaring war on the virus?

It was hard to grasp, but Hessius thought one reasonable goal was to avoid 'unnecessary deaths'. For example: if a young guy flips over his new Volvo, he shouldn't be faced with an overburdened hospital with all ICU beds taken.

There was another important thing to achieve: nurses, doctors, and all other hospital staff needed to dare go to work.

This was really nothing strange: identify the crisis, find out what can go wrong, and make sure to maintain important functions. These were things that most middle managers were taught in a weekend at some boring conference centre.

So what was the most cost-effective way to achieve these goals?

The two economists by her side shifted uneasily in their seats. That was no way to talk. Not now. Not while people were dying.

Afterwards, the irritation continued to mount inside Hessius. At the same time, she started to hesitate. This was apparently more controversial than she'd thought.

During these weeks in March, as Europe shut down its societies and economies, it was said on several occasions that no expenses would be spared. This was war. You couldn't put a price on people's lives.

But the economic sciences had spent decades, centuries, doing just that: putting a price on people's lives.

In several cases, it had happened before it was even called economics. Remember Daniel Bernoulli, who calculated the societal gains of vaccinating a whole population against smallpox? If you ask a true economic believer, they'll even tell you it's possible to save lives by calculating with lives.

One story often told begins with a flight from Denver to Chicago in 1989. One of the engines exploded at 37,000 feet, and the pilots brought the plane down for an emergency landing.

On the plane were four babies. They didn't have their own seats; instead, they sat on their parents' laps. So the flight attendants told the parents to place the babies on the floor — in complete accordance with the rules of the time. As the plane struck the ground in Iowa, it broke apart and caught on fire. More than 100 people died — among them, one of the children who hadn't been strapped in.

After the accident, many demanded that the world's aviation authorities change their rules, so that little children had to be strapped in, in their own seats. Several organisations — among them, the American Academy of Pediatrics and the American National Transportation Safety Board — supported the demands. For why should the smallest children enjoy less protection than other passengers?

But it wasn't that simple. When economists began to calculate what would happen if all parents were forced to buy tickets for their infants, they discovered something worrying. Some travellers would take the car instead. And as it was considerably more dangerous to travel by car than by aeroplane, more children would die.

Doing nothing would save lives.

Statistical lives versus real lives. Lives now versus future lives. These were the things Kerstin Hessius had on her mind as she continued to work from home.

In the apartment, her husband paced back and forth with his phone glued to his ear. He worked for a company that owned hotel properties, and, judging by the half of the conversations she could hear, things were going from bad to worse. The cancellations were pouring in.

People were calling her up: young entrepreneurs who'd had their funding withdrawn, people seeing their lives' work ruined.

Now upper-secondary schools had closed and transitioned to remote learning. So had universities. The government said it might become necessary to close schools for younger children, too.

Kerstin Hessius had a flashback to when she graduated university at the beginning of the 1980s. There was a recession in Sweden, and no one knew when it was going to end.

It was complete and utter darkness, she remembered.

Now, the darkness had returned.

She felt ill at ease. Why was no one addressing what was happening? You couldn't just strip young people of their future. Why didn't anyone have the guts to speak up?

Then she was struck by an idea. Perhaps there was no one in all of Sweden more suited than her? After all, she was responsible for a not-inconsiderable portion of the Swedish people's future prosperity, and she had a platform.

She got out her notes from the failed discussion with the other economists, and wrote an article in the space of a few hours. Then she called *Svenska Dagbladet*.

A cancelled debate

On the morning of 20 March, Johan Giesecke was gearing up. He had an important match later that evening. It wasn't a title match, no. After all, it wasn't Neil Ferguson he'd be facing off against in a debate. The person who'd be standing across from him in Sweden's Television's studio just after nine o'clock that evening would be Ferguson's Swedish incarnation — Joacim Rocklöv.

Giesecke had a good feeling about this. He'd perused Rocklöv's report — the one warning that the Swedish healthcare system was on the brink of collapse — and found several errors. Eight, as a matter of fact.

This was going be fun.

At the Public Health Agency, attitudes toward Rocklöv were frosty, to say the least. Anders Tegnell thought the boy from Umeå had plagiarised the Imperial report and presented a nightmare scenario that was of no use to anyone right now.

Initially, the agency had tried to play Rocklöv down in a few subtle ways. When he sent his first piece on Covid to the agency, Lisa Brouwers didn't reply. When Rocklöv asked whether they'd received his email, she wrote back curtly, saying they didn't read unreviewed manuscripts.

This wasn't true. Both she and Anders Tegnell had looked over and discussed several unpublished studies.

Tom Britton, on the other hand, didn't quite understand why they hated Rocklöv so. When the agency sent one of its own reports to Britton, he immediately noticed they had left out Rocklöv's latest study.

Britton emailed back and told them they had to include both Rocklöv and Imperial among their references. For 'political' reasons, if nothing else.

'Failing to mention the foremost international group and the most serious Swedish publication so far gives the impression that you haven't lifted your gaze to see what others are doing.'

They really didn't like Rocklöv.

The feeling was mutual. Even though Rocklöv had never worked with the Public Health Agency — mostly, instead, with the ECDC and Imperial College — he'd begun to feel a rising irritation at the icy response from the capital.

Five days earlier, he had met Anders Tegnell for the first time.

During these weeks, the country's epidemiologists, infectious-disease doctors, and politicians would typically encounter each other in one of the waiting or makeup rooms at Sweden's Television.

It was ahead of a broadcast of the social affairs program *Agenda*, late on Sunday 15 March, that Tegnell and Rocklöv had met. Also in the room were the minister for financial markets, Per Bolund, and the former minister for finance Anders Borg.

Tegnell did most of the talking. He explained to the two politicians why the spread in Wuhan had dropped so abruptly. It wasn't because the Chinese had cracked down on the virus with force, Tegnell argued, but because the city had reached herd immunity.

That's not at all clear, Rocklöv thought, but didn't say anything at the time.

Now, not even a week had passed since their brief encounter, but a lot had happened: Imperial had presented its report, Denmark and Norway had closed their schools, and Rocklöv had come out with his alarming calculations.

Two distinct alternatives were beginning to crystallise. Close down society? Or wait?

But Anders Tegnell wouldn't be the one defending the Swedish line against the attack from Umeå. This was about scientific modelling, so Tegnell had asked Johan Giesecke if he wanted to do the debate.

Giesecke had said yes. That Friday afternoon, he carried around his list of eight erroneous assumptions, waiting to leave for the TV building.

But around 5.30 pm, Giesecke received an update. Immediately, he sat down in front of his computer and wrote to Anders Tegnell, Lisa Brouwers, Tom Britton, Jan Albert, and a few others.

'Hi everyone. They just called from [Sweden's Television] and told me Rocklöv is cancelling. He "wants to wait until the study is reviewed and ready". Wise of him. And my guess is that'll be the last we hear of that study.'

Giesecke had won in a walkover.

'Good news,' Brouwers wrote back.

'Good work Johan,' wrote Tegnell.

Giesecke wanted to suggest one more thing: wasn't it time to end the email chain with the subject line 'Imperial College' now?

The price tag

Instead of there being a debate between Joacim Rocklöv and Johan Giesecke, Kerstin Hessius ended up standing alone, with a glass of water, in front of an oval-shaped table in Sweden's Television's studio on the evening of 20 March.

It had only been 24 hours since her article was published online. That morning, an excerpt had been included in the print edition.

'We must immediately halt the actual disaster we are in, which is even worse than the potential disaster we are trying to avoid.'

That's how the article ended.

Her opinions were unique from an international perspective as well. In no other country had anyone in her position had the guts to convey the same message.

Throughout the day, the country's movers and shakers — from the minister for finance and the leader of the opposition to the head of the Swedish Trade Union Confederation — had now been forced to answer what they thought about the 'price tag for stopping the coronavirus'. It put them in a rather awkward spot.

Kerstin Hessius hadn't just turned the debate on its head. She'd lit it on fire with a Molotov cocktail. And she'd brought a few cans of jet fuel to the TV studio that evening. Now, she was relaying a sped-up, sharpened, almost Joycean 'stream-of-consciousness' version of what she'd written in the *Svenska Dagbladet* article: Are there any issues where we only study the problem without analysing the consequences of our interventions ... there have to be more efficient ways of limiting the risk of overcrowding hospitals than shutting down the whole economy, that should go without saying, really ... a whole generation is about to lose their future if this doesn't stop immediately ... why aren't the politicians doing anything about it?

Two other people were also standing at the table, but they didn't get many words in during the minutes-long conversation.

'Isn't it cynical to weigh human lives against the economy?' the moderator tried to suggest.

'No! These are not economic effects. This is not about economics, it's about people!'

Once again: statistical lives versus real lives. Lives now versus future lives.

Perhaps there was no other country in the world as receptive to the idea of statistical lives as Sweden. Perhaps there was no country closer to Daniel Bernoulli's cold calculations about human lives.

As early as 1749, the numbers-focused Swedes had begun to publish population statistics through what was then known as the Table Commission. It was the start of what would become the world's longest continuous set of population data. During the two centuries that followed, this passion for numbers mingled with economic theories, social engineering, and Keynesian arrogance, finally deteriorating into a form of technocratic hubris.

In the 1960s, the Swedish Road Administration began to use something known at the time as CBA. It was short for cost-benefit analysis, and consisted of calculations meant to help the agency choose which projects to build. A new highway bridge outside Malmö or a central barrier between Gävle and Sandviken? A widening of route 111 or of route 73?

As it was the citizens' money, various research projects were initiated to ask Swedes about their priorities. Safety or accessibility? And so on.

These methods quickly found their way into the healthcare system. By setting a price on a 'quality-adjusted life year' — a QALY — the authorities developed a method for deciding which treatments and medications to pay for.

In the 2000s, when Anders Tegnell, as head of the unit for infectious-disease control at the National Board of Health and Welfare, decided to start vaccinating Swedish girls — but not boys — against the oncogenic virus HPV, it was justified with reference to the cost per QALY for the girls at US$50,000, while the cost per QALY for vaccinating the boys would come in at more than $120,000.

The overarching approach was criticised every now and then — by both Swedes and foreigners — long before the Chinese virus began to spread. The specific models were questioned, too. But most of the time, it simply led the models to become even more complex.

When Barack Obama's big healthcare reform was being debated in the US in 2009, the Republican governor Sarah Palin coined the term 'death panels'. She pictured the consequence of increased government influence as bureaucrats deciding whether a patient 'deserved care'.

There were no bureaucrat panels in Obamacare, aside from a small detail granting families of Medicare patients voluntary counselling about end-of-life care — a passage later cut from the bill. But if Sarah Palin had been describing the workings of the Swedish healthcare system, she wouldn't have been too far off.

To this day, it is in large part bureaucrats who decide which patients deserve care in Sweden. And Swedes seem to think that's fine.

Kerstin Hessius was anxious about how her opinions would be received. And she wasn't alone. After the Sweden's Television segment on 20 March, the team at the Third National Pension Fund provided her with a small security detail. No one knew how people would react.

The day after, Hessius got her answer.

The clip spread on social media. The next day, for the first time in her life, she was recognised in the supermarket. After appearing for four minutes on national television, Hessius went from being a public figure to a celebrity.

There was no storm of people who thought she wanted to sacrifice the elderly on the altar of the market. Leif Östling, former CEO of the truck manufacturer Scania, said she was living in a 'finance bubble'. But most people who got in touch were pleased.

It was as though Swedes had been collectively reminded of their own priorities — of the society they had built. Many who reached out were grateful she'd had the guts to be so outspoken.

But most grateful were perhaps the people running the country.

On Sunday 22 March, Kerstin Hessius once again found herself in a crowded makeup room in the Sweden's Television building on Gärdet in Stockholm. She had been there so many times she had got to know the makeup artists.

Suddenly, she heard a familiar voice. She looked up.

'Who have we here?'

It was Ibrahim Baylan, the Social Democrat who had been part of Stefan Löfven's government since the 2014 shift in power. He had served as minister for energy, minister for government coordination, and — for little over a year now — minister for business, industry, and innovation.

All heads turned before Baylan continued, his eyes on Hessius.

'It's our hero.'

A balancing act

It wasn't so strange that Hessius's gesticulating in the TV studios had been met with appreciation by the ministers jointly governing the country.

With each passing day, the rest of the world introduced even stricter measures, and the atmosphere grew increasingly frantic. With each passing day, the Swedish strategy became even more exceptional.

On 23 March, the United Kingdom fell in line. That day, the British government issued a stay-at-home order and, without taking a vote, the House of Commons approved an emergency law giving the government powers it hadn't had since the end of the Second World War.

The country's media reacted neither to the shift in the balance of power, nor to the restrictions on people's liberties. Instead, Prime Minister Boris Johnson was criticised for having acted too late. An editorial in *The Times* compared Johnson to Neville Chamberlain — Winston Churchill's predecessor, considered by historians to have waited too long to quell the power-hungry ambitions of Nazi Germany.

In Sweden, the debate looked very different. Thanks to the outlier position taken by Kerstin Hessius, the Public Health Agency — and the government — suddenly found themselves on some kind of middle ground, in some form of balance.

On Tuesday 24 March, the leaders of the seven Swedish parties represented in parliament — plus one colleague each — joined a Zoom call with the prime minister.

On the call, Stefan Löfven explained the balance between different social interests that the Public Health Agency was trying to maintain.

'The fundamental focus is of course on fighting the virus and protecting people's lives and health.'

At the same time, he said, the government needed to introduce measures to limit the impact on Sweden's economy.

'Then the difficulty is that these measures will be in conflict with each other.'

The parliamentary situation in the country was complicated, to say the least. The two parties in government — the Social Democrats and the Green Party — would collaborate with the Centre Party and the Liberals on a number of issues, primarily concerning the budget. The four remaining parties formed the opposition: a motley parliamentary crew consisting of the Left Party, the Moderates, the Christian Democrats, and the Sweden Democrats.

But so far, there were no apparent differences between the opinions of the government, the semi-opposition, and the opposition. These three groups were largely in agreement on the balance in society. They all bobbed somewhere near the middle of the waterway whose navigation marks were the respective positions of Kerstin Hessius and Emmanuel Macron.

Stefan Löfven explained that the government was prepared to make more decisions if there was a formal request from the Public Health Agency. This triggered the resumption of a discussion initiated the previous Tuesday — about whether the government should really be sitting around waiting for requests from the agency, or if it ought to prepare additional measures of its own.

The prime minister seemed to think the discussion presupposed an opposition that didn't exist.

'I think the authorities are very clear about the focus being to protect the elderly and at-risk groups. And that is also what the government has signalled. We're not handing over everything to the authorities.'

The gym and the cookie jar

The European Centre for Disease Prevention and Control had a view overlooking both an eight-lane highway and the Royal Palace's expansive Haga Park.

It was a relatively new institution. After the SARS outbreak in 2003, the bureaucrats in Brussels had sped up their plans for a European infectious-disease agency. Like most projects the union undertook, it had quickly deteriorated into a tug of war between member states about where the agency should be located. After all, there were many jobs involved.

It was partly thanks to Johan Giesecke that it ended up in the Swedish capital. First, he'd run around the corridors of the Government Offices, lobbying for Sweden to apply. Then he'd fought those who, for reasons of regional policy, wanted to situate the agency somewhere other than Stockholm.

And, finally, he'd ascended the throne as the newly formed agency's first chief scientist.

Since 2014, that post had been held by a Brit named Mike Catchpole.

Catchpole went to a gym. It was run by the Norwegian company SATS, but it had been closed because of the pandemic. The publicly listed chain had closed all its gyms in Sweden, Norway, and Finland on 12 March.

But on 23 March, a cheerful message popped up in Catchpole's inbox. 'We're re-opening,' it said. 'Welcome!'

In its message, SATS referred to the Swedish Public Health Agency's recommendations.

Catchpole was perplexed. He reached out to Anders Tegnell. Could this really be true?

It was. The next day, the agency sent out a media release with the headline 'Go Work Out but Do So Safely'.

'Physical activity is good for public health,' it said. 'Sports and exercise should therefore continue.'

* * *

Of the 271 people working at the ECDC, around three-quarters had migrated from the rest of Europe. These foreign officials and scientists were like paratroopers airdropped into the small Scandinavian country, and now they were greatly surprised at the way their temporary home country was handling the crisis facing the world.

A few of them tried to conduct small personal crusades against this perceived indifference. One employee even emailed their child's preschool, demanding that it shut down.

It didn't.

Over the past two weeks, Catchpole had watched with his own eyes as Sweden diverged from the other European countries.

And now his gym was about to open its doors again?

It wasn't just officials at the EU infectious-disease agency who were surprised at the Swedish approach. Most people who knew anything about the country were just as baffled.

Up until the spring of 2020, the image of Sweden in the rest of the world had remained the same as in the past few decades: here was a well-organised, boring welfare state. Swedes were 'Germans dressed up as human beings', as the Danes liked to say.

Anyone taking a guided tour at the National Museum in Copenhagen might even be offered a condensed explanation of why Swedes had become so uncool: they'd been subjected to a much stricter version of Martin Luther's teachings. In Denmark, it was said, the congregation was more important than the Bible. In Denmark, the priest didn't come into people's homes and interrogate them about their knowledge of the Bible and Luther's Small Catechism.

Swedes were much more bound by rules. How else to explain their strict drug laws and the fact that they always wore bicycle helmets, were forced to buy their alcohol from special state-run shops, and built roundabouts everywhere?

When authors described Swedish society, they would sometimes claim that it had been overcome by something like a panic disorder. Like a patient seeing threats in anything that could be dangerous but rarely was, Sweden had an excessive need for safety and control.

'Zero tolerance' and 'zero vision' were distinctively Swedish terms. They were used across both traffic and drug policy. No one should have to die in a car — no one should be taking drugs.

Over the years, Swedish politicians at all levels had proposed — and often managed to pass — zero-tolerance plans for bullying, drowning, suicides, unemployment, as well as radon in people's homes.

And yet, with Sweden so close by, the Danes knew it wasn't just a classroom governed by prefects. The classic counterexample was the fact that it was illegal to jaywalk in Denmark, but not in Sweden.

Moreover, since the 1990s, Swedish society had been caught up in a swift liberalisation. Everything from its school system to immigration policy lay closer to a neoliberal dream state than to a European social-democratic party platform.

But that hadn't changed the world's image of Sweden.

They seemed to be a cautious people.

At the beginning of March, when the Public Health Agency began to invite journalists to the northern parts of the Swedish capital, where Stockholm seamlessly gives way to Solna, everything changed.

It all started with a cookie jar.

Outside the press room where the daily briefings were being held was a spartan table of refreshments: a coffee thermos, a pitcher of tap water, some plastic mugs — and a tin jar.

The jar contained stale Swedish butter cookies. A few journalists plunged their fists into the jar and fished out a couple of cookies. Others looked on, wide-eyed. A dangerous virus was sweeping across the world — and the government agency in charge of protecting the Swedish people hadn't even thought to provide a spoon?

A week later, Anders Tegnell took a Danish journalist out to lunch in the agency's cafeteria.

'The buffet is delicious,' the state epidemiologist said.

Another Danish journalist — from the newspaper *Information* — looked on in surprise: 'Seen from Denmark, it was almost like diving into an episode of German *Big Brother*. You almost expected the state epidemiologist to invite the journalist to sip champagne from his bellybutton.'

Tegnell's boss — Johan Carlson — also seemed unfazed by the pandemic. Every day, he commuted from his home in Uppsala by train, Metro, and bus. He even let the local paper follow along on a trip to work. When he went to restaurants, other guests looked at him in surprise.

But most extreme was Johan Giesecke. He gladly informed the papers that he saw his grandchildren often. He went on TV several times a week. When someone asked him how he could be doing these things despite having turned 70, he replied: 'I usually say I'm 69.'

Tegnell received letters from people who were furious. How could Giesecke be allowed to go on TV night after night when, according to the agency's own guidelines, he was supposed to self-isolate?

In just a few weeks, these three men alone managed to change a century-old image of Sweden.

The strategy taken by the small country had many names in the foreign press: 'Laissez-faire strategy', 'Take-it-on-the-chin approach', 'Russian roulette strategy'. There were many ways to describe this contempt for death.

For anyone with knowledge of the history of infectious-disease control in Sweden, the choice seemed even more surprising.

Sweden's strictness was a chapter of its own in medical history. The quarantine law introduced in the country as early as 1806, after an outbreak of yellow fever, had been characterised by historians as 'furious'. Sea captains on ships violating its provisions could be put to death. Suspected vessels had to dock at Känsö, outside Gothenburg, and patients were forced to shave their heads and have their bodies washed in vinegar.

A few decades later, in 1853, smallpox vaccination became mandatory in Sweden. While other countries in Europe balanced the state's needs against the free will of its citizens, it wasn't until 1916 that Swedish parents were given any opportunity to except their children from vaccination.

In the fight against sexually transmitted diseases, the Swedish state clamped down with equal force. Requirements that were imposed only on sex workers in other countries were applicable to the entire Swedish population. A law named 'Lex Veneris' was passed in 1918, meaning that any person infected with a sexually transmitted disease was obliged to seek medical attention and participate in treatment and contact tracing.

The Swedish system garnered great interest abroad. The New York City mayor Fiorelli LaGuardia was impressed, and in 1935 he sent a committee to suss out whether anything they were doing there could be replicated. But the resulting report was criticised by *The Lancet*: the Swedish policy wasn't the way to go. Having to answer questions about who could have spread the disease was considered deeply offensive, and stigmatising, to people.

Others piled on. British authorities at this time considered contact tracing a fascist means of control, proven by the fact that it was practised in both Italy and Germany.

Sweden's hardline strategy was still going strong when the world went through the HIV epidemic of the 1980s. Once again, Sweden stood out as an exceptionally harsh country. As one of very few democratic states, Sweden allowed the forced isolation of individuals infected with HIV.

Now — in 2020 — the country had moved to the other end of the spectrum. Its public-health paternalism, safety addiction, and somewhat 'fascist' measures of infectious-disease control had been replaced by extreme liberty.

What had happened?

A few of the researchers who had followed the history of infectious-disease control in Sweden ventured a guess that perhaps this historical strictness was the cause. In the decades that had passed since the HIV epidemic, the hard line had been hashed over in books and TV shows, as well as in legal and historical dissertations. Society seemed to have reached a consensus that politicians and infectious-disease specialists had gone too far.

Was that why the hard line had been exchanged for its opposite?

The controversial cookie jar was eventually removed and replaced with candy that was carefully wrapped, if perhaps somewhat hard to chew.

At the press conferences where the candy was handed out, Anders Tegnell tried to hammer home the message that Sweden wasn't so different from other countries. The big distinction, he said, was that the Swedish measures were voluntary. So even though they'd had few decrees from their decision-makers, the Swedish people had reduced their activity significantly.

There was a large grain of truth in that description. Once the agency recommended that Stockholmers work from home, the central, office-dominated parts of the capital had been transformed into a ghost town.

The effects of social distancing — the awkward, misleading concept that should really have been called *physical* distancing — could be seen in various ways. The annual winter vomiting bug ceased abruptly; cases of seasonal influenza were dropping fast.

But the difference between Sweden and other countries was visible to the naked eye. While states in the US were issuing one stay-at-home order after another, while the Belgian police monitored their parks with drones, while Germans and Brits were allowed to gather in groups of no more than two, Swedes continued to go to spin classes, drink beer in bars, and take ski trips to the mountains.

Now the most famous tourist town in the Swedish mountain range — Åre — was nicknamed 'the next Ischgl' by the German newspaper *Süddeutsche Zeitung*. Typically, when a destination in Sweden was adorned with the adjective 'next' in the foreign press, this was good news for the Swedish hospitality industry. But the analogy to the Austrian ski town had nothing to do with an extensive lift system or exciting off-piste opportunities. Instead, it suggested that the northern Swedish municipality now risked becoming a Covid-19 epicentre of the same proportions as Ischgl had been a few weeks earlier.

Compared to several European countries, the Swedish death toll remained low. For this reason, there was still something both foreboding and admonishing about the media coverage.

But, so far, the Swedish authorities chose not to heed the warnings.

The company SkiStar, which owned several ski resorts across Sweden and Europe, had been forced to close its resorts in St Johann, Austria, and Trysil, Norway — but was still keeping its Swedish destinations open.

Regardless of what Anders Tegnell was trying to argue in the daily press conferences, it was becoming increasingly clear both to Swedes and to the outside world that Sweden had, in fact, chosen a very different path.

This raised the stakes significantly for both the government and the Public Health Agency.

Screwing up in the company of others is rarely a problem. Screwing up on your own, however, is an entirely different matter.

On 25 March, the most widely read political commentator in the country — Viktor Barth-Kron at *Expressen* — wrote that both the Public Health Agency and the government were playing a dangerous game.

'Either we come out of this crisis in better shape than comparable countries, or at least not worse. If so, Anders Tegnell is set to become the new Hans Rosling, and Stefan Löfven will look to be the coolest prime minister in Europe — the one who achieved the best outcome per effort, causing the least injury to both the economy and individual liberties in proportion to what was achieved.

'Or Sweden will do worse than its more restrictive neighbouring countries. If so, to put it mildly, a very different debate awaits.'

That day, the media reported that a total of 42 Swedes had died.

'It provides a somewhat bleak picture'

On 25 March, Neil Ferguson testified before the Science and Technology Committee in the UK parliament. Among other things, he said that the British healthcare apparatus would be able to weather the storm of Covid patients, and that the death toll would come in below 20,000 people.

The magazine *New Scientist* ran a commentary on his testimony, which was subsequently quoted in a Twitter thread by the journalist and lockdown sceptic Alex Berenson.

That thread, in turn, was pasted into an email from Jan Albert to both Johan Giesecke and Anders Tegnell. The subject line read: 'Ferguson makes a U-turn?'

'Interesting!' Giesecke replied.

'For sure,' wrote Tegnell.

Anyone reading the original testimony would have had a hard time finding evidence of Ferguson changing his position — even less to support his making a 'U-turn'. But the enthusiasm in Solna was telling in the last week of March.

A lot of things seemed to be going the Swedish public servants' way.

The curve showing the number of new intensive-care patients looked flat — a lot flatter than in other countries. Tegnell said the situation 'remained serious', but also that the increase in hospitalisations was happening 'relatively slowly'. The healthcare system seemed ready, too. It was 'as prepared as it could be', according to Tegnell.

'This looks so very different from what we've seen in many of the countries that have truly struggled,' he said to TT News Agency on Sunday 29 March.

The agency's image had improved, too. The foreign media had begun to take a different kind of interest in the Swedish strategy. Flower deliveries were pouring into Anders Tegnell's office and home.

In the email threads, they also noted that deaths in Lombardy were reaching a plateau at around 5,000.

The question was why. Was it the lockdowns that were halting the deaths? Or was this a more permanent mortality figure due to herd immunity?

Johan Giesecke felt it was time to lift some of the restrictions that had been introduced. On 27 March, he emailed Anders Tegnell and Johan Carlson, suggesting that upper-secondary schools and universities be allowed to return to in-person teaching. The epidemiological value of keeping students at home was non-existent. Besides, it would be a signal that brighter days were coming.

'I feel especially sorry for everyone currently in their [final year] — it's a shame not to get to celebrate one's graduation after 12 years at school.'

By now, around 200 Swedish deaths due to Covid-19 had been reported. That figure could be interpreted in several ways. So far, the death toll wasn't remarkably high compared to that of, say, Italy. But, at the same time, the Swedish curve was beginning to tick upward compared to those of its Nordic neighbours.

On the evening of Sunday 29 March, Tom Britton sent around a new model he had been working on. It simulated the spread of infection among the 2 million people living in what he called Greater Stockholm.

Among the recipients were Anders Tegnell, Johan Giesecke, and Jan Albert.

'It provides a somewhat bleak picture,' he wrote.

For a mathematician, knowing the infection fatality rate, or the share of infected people who died, was valuable. Slowly, an unknown variable in the equations began to be replaced by actual numbers.

Now he could reverse-engineer the scenario. He already knew the number of people who had died from Covid; that was reported in the news every day. With his guesstimate of how many infected Swedes it took to kill one Swede, he could calculate how many Swedes had been infected so far. No one knew for certain how high the infection fatality rate was, but that variable, too, was becoming less uncertain with each passing day. The way Britton interpreted the literature, the mortality measures were being steadily adjusted downward.

He now assumed an infection fatality rate of 0.3 per cent.

So he divided 200 by 0.003, and rounded up the numbers.

Sixty-seven thousand — that's how many people might have been infected in early March.

There were many uncertainties involved. The timeframe of three weeks may just as well have been 2.5 or 3.5 weeks. And the infection fatality rate could be 0.15 or 0.6 per cent.

Yet the picture remained bleak.

Moreover, those 67,000 infected people — whether there were a little more or a little fewer — had been waltzing around the capital unrestricted for some time. In Britton's model, as in the real world, restrictions had only been introduced from the middle of March.

They had taken the Metro, gone shopping, travelled by bus.

Now, Tom Britton's guess was that between 15,000 and 20,000 Swedes would die before the epidemic was over.

'Naturally, I won't be sharing this with anyone other than yourselves,' Britton ended his email.

At nine in the evening, Tegnell replied: 'Mulling this over and letting Lisa have a look.'

When he was interviewed by the media, Anders Tegnell continued to sound optimistic. Things were quietening down, he said.

But beneath the surface, a degree of uncertainty had begun to take root.

'The next three weeks will be terrible'

On 5 April, Johan Giesecke emailed Anders Tegnell, Lisa Brouwers, and Tom Britton.

He wanted to let them know about a French professor. This professor had once been head of the preparedness unit at the ECDC. Like Giesecke, he had retired, and, like Giesecke, he had nevertheless continued to work with unflagging intensity. This professor hadn't even bothered to leave Sweden. He loved to go sailing in the Baltic, and his wife still worked at the ECDC.

From his home, the professor monitored diseases, drew charts, and wrote analyses. Overall, he had many interests. The most obscure was his interest in traffic signs; he collected photographs of crosswalks from different countries, and had at one time exhibited them in a gallery in Stockholm.

The professor's name was Denis Coulombier — that is, the same Coulombier who a month previously had marched into the Public Health Agency to personally warn Anders Tegnell of the new virus.

But Johan Giesecke knew nothing of that.

Giesecke admired Coulombier's abilities, not least the Frenchman's 'broad, lateral thinking'.

'He's one of the five most intelligent people I know,' he wrote in his email to Tegnell, Brouwers, and Britton.

A few hours later, Britton replied: 'Johan speaks of an acquaintance who is one of the five most intelligent people he knows. Very flattering to be on the recipients' list, then! I can only interpret this to imply that we are the other four.'

Giesecke replied: 'Sorry, Tom. You're good, but I'm keeping the identities of the other four to myself.'

Giesecke continued the email with a detailed recounting of a scene from the film *Cincinnati Kid*. In it, Steve McQueen loses a game of poker to an ageing master.

Giesecke quoted the master (almost) verbatim: 'You are good, Kid. You are very good. But as long as I'm around you'll only be second best.'

Then Giesecke added: 'To avoid any misunderstanding I would like to emphasise that I don't count myself among those five. Watch the film — it's good.'

But one of those five people was Denis Coulombier. And now he and Anders Tegnell made contact once more.

The Frenchman and the state epidemiologist soon started squabbling over some data. One issue concerned the measure of movement in society. Like a mantra, the Public Health Agency was repeating the line that Swedes had reduced their travelling as much as other nationalities had — despite not being forced to do so by government decisions or hastily written laws. It showed, Tegnell argued, that recommendations sufficed to get people to limit their contacts.

The question was whether this was true.

Coulombier sent the agency statistics from Google. The American tech giant's business idea had long been to gather as much data as possible on its users — and then to exploit that information to sell as closely targeted ads as possible.

During the Covid-19 pandemic, this information gained new value. By measuring how much citizens moved around, it was possible to see what impact the advice, recommendations, laws, and decrees about avoiding social contacts were having.

For a few weeks, the company had been compiling so-called mobility reports that professional and amateur epidemiologists could use to observe people's movement patterns.

Coulombier sent the figures for the previous weekend, from 3 to 5 April. They showed that Sweden had the lowest reduction — at only 7 per cent. Spain and Italy, by comparison, had reduced their movements in society by more than 66 per cent.

But Tegnell had different figures. The Swedish telecom provider Telia was allowing the Public Health Agency free access to a service it called Telia Crowd Insights. And it showed a much more significant decrease.

'We're getting better data from Telia showing that mobility in Sweden has diminished markedly,' came Tegnell's short reply.

The analysis sent by Coulombier to Giesecke on 5 April, and which later ended up with Tegnell, differed on one crucial point from the agency's and Britton's calculations.

While Britton and the Public Health Agency believed that Sweden was already at the peak of transmission, in Coulombier's calculation that point lay two weeks into the future. And the peak for new deaths was three weeks away.

Because the number of infections as well as deaths was increasing exponentially, those weeks would make a big difference.

'In the space of one week, the number of deaths will at least quadruple,' Coulombier wrote to Giesecke before ending his email: 'Have a nice Sunday. The next three weeks will be terrible.'

Part IV

Antibodies

From the northern shore of Kungsholmen in Stockholm, just opposite Karlberg Castle, two jetties reach out into the narrow section of Lake Mälaren that connects the Riddarfjärden waters to a bay called Ulvsundasjön.

One day in April, Åke Lundkvist headed there.

The sounds from the marinas were a sure sign that spring was arriving in the Swedish capital. As the days grew longer, enthusiasts began to scrape away flaking paint, fix up dodgers, and oil wooden components ahead of summer.

Stockholm's waters were surprisingly empty for this time of the year. The launching had been delayed because of new rules about which bottom paints were allowed. Around the city, boat owners were still blasting their hulls.

If you could have seen Lundkvist on his way to the marina, with his black leather jacket, lean body, and beautifully furrowed face, you would have struggled to guess that he was a professor of molecular virology. He looked more like the guitarist in some band that had seen its heyday in the 1980s but still went on tour.

Lundkvist owned a wooden boat he used to cruise around in on Lake Mälaren. Sometimes he'd take it through a lock into the bay of the Baltic Sea known as Saltsjön. But he wasn't here to take his boat out or to blast the hull. Not today.

He was here to search for antibodies.

The human immune system is one of the most complex apparatuses in the world. The way in which our bodies fight pathogens began to develop almost 500 million years ago. We have a clue about this because certain animals that existed back then — such as sharks — in some sense have the same immunological operating system as us.

That's a very crude simplification. But the timespan gives you an idea of the work required today to identify all the little details and functions that exist; evolution has had a long time to work on the immune system.

The number of diseases and ailments that may in some way be connected to the immune system — from MS, diabetes, AIDS, and rheumatism to common allergies and eczema — are further signs of an untold complexity.

The scientist who did the most to shape our image of the immune system was the German Paul Ehrlich. Towards the end of the nineteenth century — when the world's doctors had come around to the theory that viruses and bacteria were the cause of many diseases — he tried to answer one basic question: how does the body know which viruses and bacteria to attack?

His solution was strongly influenced by the technology of the era. Ehrlich was captivated by a new scientific method making it possible to dye tissue in animals and people. If, for instance, you injected methylthioninium chloride — or methylene blue — into an animal, it seemed to travel towards the nervous system. Perhaps there was something in the body that travelled towards a parasite or other intruder in the same way and destroyed it?

Paul Ehrlich had a theory. When something that didn't belong entered the body — it didn't have to be bacteria, it might also be a poison — certain kinds of cells rushed out.

These cells carried little 'keys' or, rather, keychains. They fitted — well, like keys into a lock — on a part of the foreign organism. When the body was invaded by an infection, lots of these keys were produced.

The keys were given the name *antikörper* — antibodies.

It was a pretty good name. Clear, powerful, and easy to translate into lots of other languages: antibodies, *anticorps*, *anticuerpos*.

The idea behind the name was easy to grasp, too. It was no coincidence that it would go on to become one of few words from immunology to make it into common parlance.

With the help of his idea, Ehrlich could measure and quantify the way certain immune responses worked. When he injected poison into rabbits, for example, and slowly upped the dosage — to allow the rabbits to adapt — he found that they could survive doses 5,000 times stronger than levels previously thought to be lethal.

Much later, when the history of immunology was told by the author Matt Richtel in his book *An Elegant Defense,* the verdict was that Paul Ehrlich had asked precisely the right question: was there something in the body seeking out foreign viruses? The answer, however, was far more complicated than Paul Ehrlich ever thought.

But let's not go there just yet. We'll stay with antibodies for a moment.

Because the Swedish strategy was built on an assumption that the coronavirus was like an unstoppable forest fire that would sooner or later die out, the whole world soon began to take an interest in how large a part of the Swedish forest had burnt so far.

How many had actually been infected with the virus in Sweden and the rest of Europe?

One way to arrive at an answer was by conducting a so-called seroepidemiological survey. You simply selected people at random and checked their blood for antibodies against the virus. That way, you could calculate how many had undergone infection.

This kind of survey from China was what Anders Tegnell had put out a call for in the email chain about the Imperial report.

This was the 'mystery' he had spoken of.

How many people had been infected? How many had antibodies? And how high was the mortality rate?

There were some hopeful studies. On 24 March, the epidemiology professor Sunetra Gupta at the University of Oxford had, with the help of a theoretical model, come to the conclusion that more than half of all Brits had already been infected.

If the study was correct, it meant the lockdown in the UK was completely meaningless — and that Imperial College had made a wild miscalculation.

In a way, it wasn't unexpected that Oxford and Imperial would end up on opposite sides in the struggle over lockdowns. Within the world of epidemiology, the schism between the two universities was well known. It had started in 1999, when the British godfather of infectious-disease control, Roy Anderson — Sir Roy — had accused Gupta of having a fling with one of her superiors.

Sir Roy ended up having to both apologise and pay damages to

Gupta. He tried to stay at Oxford, but was eventually forced out by his colleagues.

Sir Roy then took his odds and ends and set up shop at Imperial College, where he built up the modelling unit later taken over by his protégé Neil Ferguson.

Twenty years later, Gupta and Anderson stood on opposite sides in the Covid battle. Were the countries of the world already on their way out of the epidemic — or should they remain in lockdown?

Sunetra Gupta was of the opinion that Sweden had chosen the right path through the pandemic. But so far it was all just theories — based on numbers in endless data models. As of yet, no one knew how many people had actually been infected — in Sweden or anywhere else.

Perhaps the answer was in the antibodies?

Åke Lundkvist had first met Björn Olsen 25 years before, through one of Olsen's doctoral students. They became fast friends. The pair shared the same fascination for the relationship between people, animals, and viruses. Together, they built up a zoonosis centre on Öland in the Baltic Sea and funded bird observatories.

They were both a bit contrarian. A few years earlier, they had set up a national centre for vector-borne diseases in Uppsala. The idea was to study the ecology behind infections such as borrelia, TBE, Rickettsia, and anaplasmosis. Both Lundkvist and Olsen thought the healthcare system was treating these patients badly. The problems that could linger after a TBE or borrelia infection were often hard to diagnose, which meant these people might be bounced around the primary-care system for years.

A long time ago, Anders Tegnell had been Lundkvist's boss. This was at the former Institute for Infectious Disease Control, and it had worked well. Tegnell had been more interested in policy and administration, so Lundkvist had been free to focus on his research. But when Johan Carlson took over the agency, Lundkvist had been among those who left.

What they were now doing at his old workplace was beyond Lundkvist's comprehension. He suspected the Swedish strategy had been influenced by Johan Giesecke, and more specifically by Giesecke's view of how the virus behaved.

The big difference between the Giesecke–Tegnell theory and the one that Olsen and Lundkvist believed in was the rate at which the virus spread. The former assumed the coronavirus spread like an influenza pandemic — quickly and irrepressibly, like a 'tsunami'. The latter assumed the virus's spread was significantly more protracted.

That rift between the Public Health Agency's leadership troika and the microbiologists had been growing with each passing day throughout March. Every attempt to make contact had been rejected by Tegnell.

With every step the state epidemiologist took, with every sentence he spoke, the dissenters grew stronger in their conviction that Tegnell was underqualified for his job.

Åke Lundkvist and Björn Olsen felt fairly certain that the level of immunity in society wasn't as high as the Public Health Agency thought.

They both knew how antibody testing worked. For some of the diseases on which they were experts — such as TBE — they had proved there were rapid tests that worked really well.

So, early on, the two scientists began to evaluate tests that could prove the existence of antibodies against Covid-19. They ordered hundreds of tests from nine different manufacturers across China and South Korea.

Most proved to be rather poor, but two out of the nine tests seemed promising.

Lundkvist brought one of the functioning tests to the marina. He poked some of his buddies in the fingertip and sampled their blood.

At the same time, Olsen was doing the same to his neighbours in Norra Djurgårdsstaden in Stockholm.

The rumour that Olsen and Lundkvist had acquired a bunch of antibody tests spread quickly. Lots of people wanted to find out if they'd been infected, but there was still no way for regular people to test themselves for antibodies in Sweden.

Olsen and Lundkvist passed some of the tests on to six other colleagues. Now there were eight of them administering tests among friends and acquaintances here and there across Stockholm and surrounding areas.

In just a few days, they collected 453 samples.

Åke Lundkvist compiled the results and wrote them down on a notepad.

***

Lundkvist and Olsen weren't the only ones wanting to find out what proportion of the Swedish population had been infected. In a lab at the Royal Institute of Technology in Stockholm, a researcher in measurement science named Niclas Roxhed was licking 1,000 envelopes before sending them to randomly selected people in Stockholm. The envelopes contained a small needle, a plaster, and a return envelope. The idea was for the chosen ones to prick their finger and return the sample. When what Roxhed was up to became known, he was inundated with calls from private individuals and companies wanting to know if they had been infected.

All of Stockholm seemed preoccupied with that question. At the polling company Novus, CEO Torbjörn Sjöström became so curious that he added a question to surveys otherwise focused on things such as voting preferences for political parties: 'Do you believe that you have been infected with the coronavirus?'

Johan Giesecke got involved, too. He wrote to Jan Albert wanting 10,000 tests done as quickly as possible.

Albert replied to Giesecke, saying that his colleague Matti Sällberg was almost done with a test they would be able to administer to 50,000 people. Albert suggested they start with blood donors and samples from the community testing that the Public Health Agency was already doing.

This was indispensable information. Without seroepidemiological studies, there was no knowing how many had been infected. Without that knowledge, determining the deadliness of the virus was impossible.

And if you didn't know how deadly the virus was, how could you determine what restrictions on people's lives were reasonable to stop the spread?

Soon they'd have answers.

The 22

They struck in mid-April, that many-headed body of microbiologists, mathematicians, virologists, and epidemiologists who, in email upon email, had expressed their indignation over the Public Health Agency's actions.

In an op-ed published on *Dagens Nyheter*'s website around lunchtime on 14 April, they broadcast their message: 'The Public Health Agency Has Failed — Now Politicians Must Intervene'.

The signatories were a kaleidoscopic group of people. They came from different universities around the country — from Umeå, Lund, Gothenburg. They belonged to different disciplines. But most of all, they had different relationships with the Public Health Agency.

Some — like Fredrik Elgh and Björn Olsen — harboured decade-long conflicts with Anders Tegnell, while others — like Joacim Rocklöv — had entered into their schisms quite recently.

Some were unknown to Tegnell. Others he'd had an eye on. One of the latter was Cecilia Söderberg-Nauclér, a doctor and researcher at the Karolinska Institute. She had been so loud in her criticism of the agency that Tegnell had sent Jan Albert an email with a short sentence: 'You have a problem at KI.'

The 22 signatories — who eventually came to be known simply as 'the 22' — had been sitting in video conferences late into the evening over Easter to hash out the text.

They pulled no punches. When the op-ed was finished, it was a blistering indictment of incompetence within the agency, and of cowardice among the politicians above it.

'How are we supposed to win this fight if our elected officials hide behind public servants, who have complete hold of the reins? Public servants who thus far have shown no talent for either predicting or limiting the development we are now living with.'

It wasn't entirely clear in what way the 22 signatories wanted to change the Swedish strategy. But the text mentioned that Finland —

unlike Sweden — had forced the majority of its schoolchildren to stay home, and had closed its cafés and restaurants.

It became the most read op-ed since *Dagens Nyheter* started measuring its digital reach.

In a story for Sweden's Radio about the genesis of the text, the Covid-19 pandemic was likened to a sports contest between nations. Up until then, the loyal Swedish public had supported the somewhat odd tactics of its national team in the hope that they would prove effective.

The tension had been there all along. But now it had been laid bare. Would this mark the turning point? Would the team management now be forced to change tactics? Would the manager be swapped out?

Instead, the opposite happened. Instead of a debate about Sweden's chosen path, the discussion came to focus on the article itself.

Its opening sentence mentioned the Swedish death toll. According to the 22 scientists, 10.2 people per million inhabitants had died of Covid-19 between 7 and 9 April. That figure corresponded to a daily average over those three days of 105 deaths.

When Anders Tegnell read the article, he thought these were largely the same people who always sounded the alarm as soon as a new virus started to spread around the world.

When the clock struck two that day and the daily press conference began, it was easy for him to respond to their criticism. The number of deaths cited in the article simply didn't correspond to the Public Health Agency's own figures. The death toll on those days — according to the most recent figures — had actually been between 60 and 65 per day.

'The 22' had made the mistake of studying the dates when the deaths were reported, instead of the dates on which they occurred. A large part of the reported deaths actually belonged to a backlog from the preceding weekend.

'This would never even have made it through the methodology section in an undergraduate dissertation,' a scientist at the Royal Institute of Technology wrote in the engineering trade publication *Ny Teknik*.

'An unreliable and straight-up indecent attack,' wrote an infectious-disease professor.

'The 22 scientists' reasoning is unscientific,' an ecology professor from Lund fulminated.

The 22 had indeed been guilty of a miscalculation. Yet perhaps it wasn't until they decided to write a clarification and send it to the newspaper that they truly sealed their fate. 'The figures cited, in themselves,' they wrote, 'are in our opinion less important than the fundamental development in the pandemic that we are trying to point to.'

It was a choice of words inviting an entirely new cadre of critics.

The next day, the columnist, podcaster, and author Alex Schulman wrote in *Expressen*: 'So, in plain language, what they are saying is: Sure, we were wrong, but it doesn't matter. Or, to use a familiar phrase from the land of tin foil hats: It makes no difference that it isn't true, it's still rotten.'

He went on: 'This is an intellectual meltdown. I suppose the only comfort in the face of this academic misfire is the knowledge that these 22 scientists aren't the ones behind the wheel of the country right now.'

After just a day or two, it was clear that the attack on Anders Tegnell had had a very different outcome than what was intended.

Fredrik Elgh had a Twitter account. For the header on his profile, he'd uploaded a photoshopped picture of four people among the Public Health Agency's leadership, each making an unflattering face. Behind them was a handwritten note with the words 'Virologist wanted — NB NOT Fredrik Elgh'.

When he logged on to Twitter, he could see the reactions to the text with his own eyes. It didn't look good. The 'Twitter horde', as he called it, didn't seem to care about the rest of the article. He and his fellow scientists were taunted and ridiculed. The whole thing had turned into a 'pseudo debate', he thought, about their numbers.

The question of whether or not Sweden should go into lockdown was now being turned into a proxy war between an agency and its 22 angry antagonists.

Thereby, the pressure eased — yet again — on Sweden's politicians.

The 22 scientists' exhortation — that 'our elected representatives, those who hold the overall responsibility, must step in, there is no other option' — had for the time being been nullified.

In the same way that Kerstin Hessius singlehandedly shifted the Swedish Covid debate at a sensitive stage, the op-ed had redirected it once more.

The text that had been intended to mark the start of a new strategy for Sweden had the direct opposite effect. Björn Olsen, Fredrik Elgh, Åke Lundkvist, and the others felt they were being dragged through the dirt. They were accused of fiddling with the data. They were painted as dogmatists. They appeared, quite simply, a little mad.

The wager

'Should I tell you what I really think?'

'Please.'

On 16 April, Johan Giesecke was seated in front of a traditional Swedish tile stove on his estate outside Södertälje, south of Stockholm. The spring light filtered through the window. Every now and then, he looked out through its panes at the glassy lake where he went swimming every morning, immersed in thought.

The name of the lake outside the window was Uttran. It was an elongated, slightly overfertilised body of water meandering through the municipalities of Södertälje, Botkyrka, and Salem.

Giesecke went swimming in the lake every morning, but only during the warmer half of the year. His season ended on the last day of October, regardless of the water temperature.

For a couple of weeks now, the Swedish death toll had been ticking upward — at least, according to the way it was being measured.

It was all relative. After all, it wasn't like the people who had passed away had suddenly been plucked from the Earth. Most of the people who had died in the past week had been old, sick, and frail, and would have died, if not sooner, then a few months later.

'So that's maybe not nice,' he said, in a mild Swedish accent, to the handsome Brit with whom he was speaking on Skype.

But still. This wasn't the disaster the media had decided it was.

The person Giesecke was speaking to was named Freddie Sayers, and was the executive editor of a British online magazine known as *UnHerd*. The magazine had been founded less than three years before, and, as the name implied, its journalistic concept was to offer an alternative perspective. 'To stand aside from the rest of the news pack and "to push back against the herd mentality with new and bold thinking",' read its mission statement.

A few weeks before, the *UnHerd* editorial office had started up something it was calling 'Lockdown TV'. They interviewed scientists, experts, foreign journalists, and others about the pandemic and measures being taken to combat it. So far, it hadn't been a success; their clips only had a few thousand views.

Sayers, who was half Swedish and able to read the language, had thus been able to follow the small country's lonely path through the pandemic.

For a magazine looking for alternative viewpoints, Sweden was a goldmine. And now Freddie Sayers had sunk his pickaxe into the main vein.

Johan Giesecke shared his thoughts willingly. What had happened in Sweden was that the weakest had died first, he said. As that group was thinned out, the number of new deaths would eventually drop.

In statistical terms, this was known as 'the harvesting effect', or 'mortality displacement', and it had been the subject of some discussion at the Public Health Agency.

The phenomenon could be observed after heatwaves or periods of colder temperatures, or in connection with a particularly intense seasonal flu: a period of excess mortality followed by a period of mortality deficit.

The weakest members of society were 'harvested', simply put.

Even though Johan Giesecke was particularly outspoken that day, he didn't put it in such terms. That was probably wise.

He conceded that Sweden had made its fair share of mistakes. The country should have provided better information to those who didn't speak Swedish. It should have been quicker to protect its most frail.

But anyway: it didn't matter whether societies shut down or not. The key was to protect the elderly better.

'As far as the rest of the population is concerned, we just allow it to pass through the population?' Sayers asked.

'Essentially, yes. Herd immunity.'

'How should we judge success then?' Sayers wondered.

It was now, during the hour-long interview, that Giesecke decided to tie himself to the mast. Should he tell Sayers what he *really* thought? Please.

'I almost never do this …'

But he went on: 'Some countries do this, and some countries do that

… and in the end there will be very little difference.'

Johan Giesecke said that the two of them should get together in a year's time. In exactly one year. Then they'd find that the number of deaths would be very similar.

It was as though he made a wager. There was no money at stake — only his professional honour, exposed to the world.

UnHerd had a newly started YouTube channel with less than 100,000 followers. Sayers posted the video the next day, and wrote up a summary of what Giesecke had said with 'typical Swedish bluntness'.

'That was one of the more extraordinary interviews we have done here at UnHerd.'

The interview spread across the world. Soon, more than a million people had watched it.

Johan Giesecke went from being a former state epidemiologist to a leading figure in the anti-lockdown movement that was beginning to form around the world.

The video became a talking point in conservative circles in the UK. Concerned about the extensive restrictions on people's liberties, and disappointed that they'd been introduced by one of their own — Boris Johnson — they praised the Swede's position. In the US, libertarian think tanks held up the Swedish strategy. And from Australia came reports that the conservative government feared that right-wing opinion makers now wanted a 'Swedish solution'.

These were strange bedfellows for a nation that, until just recently, had been held up by left-wing politicians as a model progressive country, with its subsidised preschools and universal healthcare.

In one of the most liked comments below the videoclip, a user calling himself 'Andy M' wrote: 'This interview defines Covid-19 for me. I've had a Swedish flag flying in my garden since week 2 of lockdown. Such an incredible, brave and confident thing for one country to do when everyone else is doing something different.'

Now the room in Giesecke's manor was transformed into an unofficial foreign ministry for the kingdom.

Through the little camera hole on his Apple computer, Johan Giesecke gave one interview after another to the foreign press. He advised governments. He guided opposition leaders. He was invited to speak about epidemic modelling before the British House of Commons.

The Swedish epidemiologist's brutal charm went viral.

As though he were the foreign minister of some big and powerful country, he even began to turn down requests. Eight conversations a day was enough.

First, he declined to speak with an opposition leader from India, but when he found out it was Rahul Gandhi — 'That's Indira Gandhi's grandchild!' — he quickly changed his mind.

He told Rahul that India shouldn't go into lockdown. Then he took a selfie in front of the screen with Gandhi's descendant.

Giesecke noticed that the attention was starting to change him. But he knew it wouldn't last forever. After all, when the pandemic was over, no one would care about him anymore.

He decided to give himself up to it. Then he'd take a break.

This would be his spring.

Dangerous opinions

If Johan Giesecke was the outspoken foreign minister of the Swedish strategy, Anders Tegnell was its head of government. His name was mentioned with increasing frequency by lockdown sceptics around the world. They were a motley crew, the people who, for one reason or another, opposed the world's lockdowns. But they were legion.

At one end of the spectrum were those who had already been critical of a society governed by experts. Many of them also questioned whether climate change was real and human-made. Among them was the British journalist and author Toby Young, who ran the site lockdownsceptics.org.

At the other end were several reputable scientists. One of them was the Stanford professor and statistics guru John Ioannidis. Fifteen years earlier, in 2005, he had shaken the entire scientific community with an article showing that, in several disciplines, any 'research finding' was more likely to be false than true.

The study — aptly named 'Why Most Published Research Findings Are False' — was the most-read scientific study ever at the *Public Library of Science*. In second and third place came 'Women's Preference for Penis Size' and 'Ten Simple Rules for Writing a Literature Review'.

Early in the pandemic, Ioannidis had written a text for the site Statnews that garnered a lot of attention. In it, he pointed out that these extensive lockdowns were based on incomplete data about how dangerous the virus really was. Like the Swedes picking apart the Imperial College report, he thought the numbers were exaggerated. The WHO's estimate of a case mortality rate of 3.4 per cent didn't just cause needless terror, it was 'meaningless'.

Belonging to the same category as Ioannidis was the 73-year-old scientist Michael Levitt. Seven years previously, he had been to Stockholm to receive the Nobel Prize in chemistry. Now, Levitt — a citizen of Israel, South Africa, the UK, and the US — was on a furious crusade against all of his governments, and a few hundred more.

He saw this as yet another example of the way his generation — after seizing all the resources on the planet and pumping its atmosphere full of carbon dioxide — was now placing another burden on coming generations.

When it came to the spread and deadliness of the virus, he made about the same analysis as Anders Tegnell and Johan Giesecke. But as he wasn't an epidemiologist, he used different language.

There appeared to be a 'saturation' point: his data showed the virus sweeping in over a country, killing the most vulnerable, and then petering out.

It was as though he baked in herd immunity with the harvesting effect, creating a whole new concept.

He guessed this saturation point would arise when a certain proportion of the population had died. Perhaps at 0.1 per cent, or a little higher. It depended largely on how old the population was.

This was a completely different theory. It might be right; it might be wrong.

The problem was that gaining traction for it was hard.

By now, a month had passed since the world had begun its lockdown experiment. A month had passed since Imperial College had presented its study.

The world had witnessed a historic event without really reflecting on it.

And the historic event wasn't actually the pandemic — we had lived through those before.

What was unique was our reaction.

The world had stopped.

But aside from the falling GDP numbers and the rising unemployment figures around the world — both official and projected — that were broadcast every now and then, no one seemed particularly interested in putting together easily deciphered figures about the lockdowns. The big media outlets of the world had put together fancy charts of the number of infections and deaths from Covid-19, but there were no journalistic products about the number of missed school days.

The world was only interested in one thing — one single figure.

No scientific output ever, Giesecke said, had had such a big impact on the world as that highly dubious study from Imperial College.

Aside from some scientists scattered around the world, few wanted — or dared — to question the reasonableness of the restrictions depriving people of their liberty.

Those who did were now finding it increasingly difficult to get their message out. When the German biostatistician Knut Wittkowski posted a video to YouTube saying that stopping an airborne or droplet-borne virus was difficult, and lockdowns were unlikely to be effective, Rockefeller University — where Wittkowski had been working for more than 20 years — sent out a press release distancing itself from his opinions.

A few days later, YouTube took down the video clip with the justification that its message went against the WHO's recommendations.

The same happened to a video titled 'The Case Against Lockdown'. It contained an interview with Michael Levitt, conducted by the journalist Toby Young.

For YouTube's parent company Alphabet — which also owned Google — this was an unusual path to take. A few years earlier, Swedish papers had published a number of articles exposing just how easily right-wing extremist and anti-Semitic content spread on the company's platforms, that the company had allowed posts containing death threats against Swedish police officers to stay up, and that a Google search of the word 'Holocaust' delivered links to propaganda claiming it never happened.

So how was it that an epidemiological debate ended up on the wrong side of free speech?

Johan Giesecke had managed to watch Wittkowski's famous YouTube clip — and agreed with his conclusions. He'd even pasted the link into an email and sent it to Tegnell.

With each passing day, Giesecke's opinions became even more politically incorrect. Now they were considered such a threat to society that they had to be censored.

For some reason, Giesecke's interviews from that spring were allowed to stay up on YouTube and other platforms — even though his message didn't notably deviate from Levitt's or Wittkowski's. Perhaps it was because of his connections to both the Swedish Public Health Agency and the WHO; it would indeed have looked peculiar if one of the WHO's own experts had been banned from YouTube for spreading a message in conflict with the organisation's recommendations.

During his audiences with journalists from different countries, Johan Giesecke sounded less and less like a retired epidemiology professor, and more like he was broadcasting radio beyond the Iron Curtain to states under totalitarian rule in Eastern Europe during the Cold War.

Instead of citing equations from his book, he quoted Winston Churchill. And when he uttered the words 'risk' or 'danger', they didn't refer to the deadliness of the virus or potential variants, but to the authoritarian tendencies he saw — in both established democracies and countries less free. China had led the way, the report from Imperial had provided lockdown policies with a scientific veneer, and now everyone else followed.

'Now, the big risk is that dark powers begin to creep up through the ground. Just look at Hungary and the dictator there.'

In that Central European country, Prime Minister Viktor Orbán had spent the previous decade building an increasingly authoritarian state. Now his government was using the pandemic crisis to further strengthen its position. Orbán had gained the right to govern Hungary by decree, and the power to set aside existing legislation, for as long as he deemed there to be a crisis. Anyone spreading information that was considered to weaken the government's defence against the coronavirus risked up to five years in prison.

The virus was dangerous. But for entirely different reasons than people thought.

'Now, everyone believes their own government is doing the right thing. It's interesting. But the feeling afterwards will be different.'

Yet Giesecke remained hopeful. People's thirst for freedom would win out in the end.

'My hope is that people will walk out when they've had enough. One police officer on the streets of Paris can catch you if you don't have a note. But when 50,000 Parisians take to the streets, the police won't be able to keep up.'

The truce

On 21 April, it was a Tuesday again. And once again the leaders of the seven parties in parliament tuned in for a meeting with the prime minister.

There had been some ruckus in the media about Zoom having poor encryption and, what's more, placing its servers in China, so now they had switched to Skype.

That day, Johan Carlson joined them, too.

Like much of the Swedish people, the country's politicians were charmed by the unaffected doctors who in the space of just a few weeks had risen to become celebrities. Some of them thought the meetings were unusually interesting. These people actually 'answered your questions', one regular participant noted. And in plain Swedish, too. This was far from the chastened, intellectually neutered heads of agencies whose tedious presentations they were usually forced to sit through.

On 21 April, Johan Carlson told the government and the party leaders about the antibody situation in Sweden.

The fog was beginning to lift. A few studies had come in — including from the Karolinska Institute — but they were based on limited, selected populations, and couldn't be generalised to the whole country.

In his assessment, it looked promising. The calculations indicated that between 20 and 30 per cent of people living in Stockholm had developed antibodies.

'We believe the immunity level in Stockholm is beginning to build up. I wouldn't be surprised if we'll be talking about 40–50 per cent here eventually. But it's significantly lower among at-risk groups.'

Isabella Lövin, the deputy prime minister and leader of the Green Party, said she was a bit concerned.

Lövin had been watching Sweden's Television the night before. Tom Britton had been in the studio to talk about his calculations. If 30 per cent of Stockholmers had now been infected, the capital would be reaching herd immunity towards the end of May.

Now Lövin wanted to know whether there was a risk that the Swedish people was being fed information that was a little *too* positive.

'That's just a small part of the country. The whole country has a long way to go.'

Carlson replied that it was a complicated question.

'That whole herd-immunity thing has gotten a little infected. I've told my colleagues we shouldn't talk so much about herd immunity as about the immunity level. In Stockholm, it's likely a situation where we have an immunity that is curbing the spread. But it varies a lot across different groups. The starting point is worse for the people we've been protecting as we emerge out of this than the people who have been up and about.'

For many of the country's politicians, the first weeks of the pandemic were a fairly pleasant time. Paradoxically, faced with the crisis, everything seemed to return to normal. The Sweden Democrats took a dive in the polls, the Social Democrats moved back towards the one-third share of voters that the party saw as its birthright, and the Moderates' share grew a little. Not by much, but enough to regain its position as Sweden's largest opposition party.

But what should they oppose?

Already, in the early days of the crisis, the Moderates had resolved not to quarrel about the epidemiological reasoning, not to go near an R_0 number, an equation, or even a lowly little antibody.

With each Tuesday-morning meeting, party leader Ulf Kristersson and his right-hand man, Per Claréus, were becoming even more certain that this was the right way to go. Those doctors seemed to have the situation under control.

Neither was the external pressure to change anything particularly high. Companies were happy with the Swedish infectious-disease strategy: schools remained open, as did shops, and consumption hadn't fallen as much as in neighbouring countries.

While the opposition in several countries criticised their governments for not having closed down society quickly or extensively enough, the Moderates initially wanted to move the window of discourse in the opposite direction. In an op-ed in *Dagens Nyheter* on 28 April, Kristersson demanded an 'exit strategy'. The government, he wrote, should 'task the Public Health Agency — together with economic experts — with establishing criteria for what developments in the virus would make it possible to begin to reopen the economy'.

But these were side notes. The resistance against the Swedish Covid strategy had no foothold in parliament — it remained extra-parliamentary, confined to scattered Facebook groups and email threads.

From Umeå, Fredrik Elgh tried to chip away at the Swedish party truce on his own. He had been politically engaged ever since the nuclear power referendum 40 years previously, and was now a stand-in candidate for the Centre Party in the Umeå Municipal Assembly.

After the 2018 election, the Centre Party had left the conservative bloc and formed a limited collaboration with the government. In its new role as a political tiebreaker, the party had gained a great deal of influence over Swedish policy.

That spring, party leader Annie Lööf was on parental leave, having been replaced by Anders W. Jonsson. He was a teacher by profession — a fact that no one had failed to notice, as the acting party leader hadn't just undergone training in handling protective equipment, but had also taken a picture of himself wearing said equipment. This picture, as well as a close-up of him wearing a stethoscope around his neck and a red doctor's tag on his chest, had subsequently been sent to *Aftonbladet*.

During the spring, Fredrik Elgh called his acting party leader several times. They talked for hours about the Swedish strategy. Elgh wanted the politicians to be tougher on the spread of the virus, but Jonsson didn't agree. The government agencies were independent, and they'd be wise to follow their strategy.

'All the parties are in agreement on that,' Jonsson said.

Elgh got nowhere. It was as though Sweden suddenly had a national unity government.

It's like in the Second World War, Elgh thought.

In their Tuesday meetings, the Moderate leader, Ulf Kristersson, usually asked the prime minister how it was going with 'the tests'.

'How are you making sure we get testing for anyone who needs it?'

'We're on it,' the prime minister replied several times.

In the beginning, it had been a technical, almost esoteric, question. The news headlines focused on the healthcare chaos in southern Europe and school closures in Denmark and Norway. Not on PCR tests and reagents.

It was just like Ulf Kristersson to geek out on a subject like that. He had spent large parts of his political career deep down in the budget tables, in low-light environments where only bureaucrats and fungi could thrive. As a former spokesperson on economic policy for the Moderates, a former municipal commissioner for social affairs in the City of Stockholm, and a former minister for social security, he had no problem spending his time in technocratic darkness. When speaking about the climate issue, he could put an entire auditorium to sleep with convoluted arguments about the vital role of hydrogen in Swedish steel production.

Kristersson read up on how countries such as Taiwan and South Korea were able to stamp out new outbreaks with intensive testing and contact tracing. In Singapore, 5,000 people — one-thousandth of the country's population — worked with contact tracing in mid-April.

The weeks went by. Perhaps those diligent countries in Asia had managed to find a middle way between panicked lockdowns — à la France, California, or Spain — and stoic calm — à la Sweden?

The East Asian way wasn't cheap. When the US Congress approved a relief bill in April, US$25 billion were set aside for testing.

But a dollar, or a Swedish krona, suddenly had a different value. The world economy was at a standstill. State budgets were being drained. Politicians who'd considered raising an excise tax by half a percentage point just a few weeks before now had to watch their bitterly earned billions disappearing down the Covid drain.

Compared to these costs, it was small change. Compared to a full-blown lockdown, the mass-testing route was cheap indeed.

'How's it going with the tests?' Kristersson asked once more.

At the Government Offices, many were annoyed at the Moderate Party leader's testing mania. They saw it as a desperate bid by Kristersson to get back in the game. He was just trying to find an angle.

It wasn't an entirely unfair characterisation. Among the top stratum of the Moderate Party, many were glad they'd finally found an issue that didn't signal open political warfare, but nevertheless had a certain relevance.

But Ulf Kristersson wasn't the only one interested in testing and contact tracing. Early in the pandemic, the head of the WHO, Tedros Adhanom Ghebreyesus himself, had said that the backbone of the world's pandemic strategy had to be a rapid scale-up of testing, contact tracing, and isolation.

'We have a simple message for all countries — test, test, test.'

Not doing so would be like attempting to 'fight a fire blindfolded'.

But Anders Tegnell and Johan Giesecke had a different view of how the fire should be fought.

Because the virus was already widespread, testing mattered less.

According to all the old theories and plans for combating pandemics, the focus of this phase, the 'pandemic phase', was on mitigating the consequences of the virus. This phase was characterised by large-scale transmission and many cases. Testing should therefore be concentrated on the healthcare services. It shouldn't be used to prevent the virus from spreading in society.

The forest was already ablaze. This they knew. Now it was a matter of clearing firebreaks — not of determining at all costs how many pines were burning in Västmanland.

The statement from the head of the WHO confounded Giesecke. He emailed his STAG — his expert group within the WHO — to ask: are we really recommending testing in the pandemic phase?

From his contacts in Asia, Giesecke received another theory about why South Korea had chosen such a peculiar path. There, parliamentary elections loomed, and this was a way for the government to show initiative.

Anders Tegnell, on the other hand, thought the world had misinterpreted the successes in East Asia.

South Korea was a good example. The country may have had an impressive testing capacity; it had been built up after the MERS outbreak a few years earlier. But the way Tegnell saw it, in South Korea the coronavirus had penetrated a delimited group. It was a large group, yet limited. By zeroing in hard on that group, the Koreans — with the help of their extensive testing capacity — had managed to get the virus under control.

In other words, South Korea had never entered the pandemic phase.

All this time, they had remained in a phase where contact tracing was meaningful.

In Sweden, as in the US, the UK, France, Spain, and many other countries, the virus had penetrated several groups at the same time. This made it much harder to carry out such targeted efforts.

And now the forest was burning.

The resistance to these new ideas took perhaps its most obvious form in the legal jujitsu Johan Carlson was practising in order to avoid having to contact-trace.

Already in late January, the agency had, for preventative purposes, asked the government to class the novel coronavirus as both a public-health hazard and a community-health hazard under the *Communicable Diseases Act*. Calling a disease a 'public' or 'community' health hazard was a bit like a court detaining someone suspected on *reasonable grounds* or *probable cause*. For most Swedish speakers, it sounded like two ways of saying the same thing, but for lawyers there was a difference. One was stronger than the other.

According to the *Communicable Diseases Act*, community-health hazards were worse.

There were plenty of diseases classed as public-health hazards: HIV, hepatitis, diphtheria, chlamydia, polio, syphilis, et cetera. But only three diseases had ever been classed as both a public- and a community-health hazard. These were Ebola, SARS, and smallpox.

Compared to these contagions, it seemed odd that '2019-nCoV', as the virus was referred to in the letter to the government, should be bestowed with such a title. But so it was.

The law was clear about the seriousness of bringing a disease within the remit of the *Communicable Diseases Act*: 'The Public Health Agency cannot limit contact tracing in the case of a public-health hazard,' it said in chapter 3, section 7.

Clear as day.

But on 26 March, Johan Carlson decided that only microbiology labs and doctors at hospitals or nursing homes would be able to report cases of the new disease.

Didn't that equate to limiting contact tracing?

Well, not quite.

Carlson found support for his approach in chapter 2, section 5 of the Communicable Diseases Ordinance. It stated: 'The Public Health Agency may announce rules on exemptions from the duty to report in relation to a particular disease.'

The Public Health Agency couldn't get away from contact tracing — but by removing the duty to report for anyone who didn't work in a lab, hospital, or nursing home, Carlson succeeded in conjuring away large amounts of reported cases.

Which meant there was a lot less to trace.

They found a loophole, Peet Tüll thought when he saw what the Public Health Agency had done.

When he'd been involved in writing the law himself, no one had taken issue with that sentence in the Communicable Diseases Ordinance — the one saying that the duty to report could be lifted for a public-health hazard. It was a little 'lapsus', Tüll confessed, but how could they have guessed that an agency would remove the duty to report for a continuing public-health and community-health hazard?

Why would anyone want to? he thought.

Johan Giesecke agreed with Tüll that they had bent the law a little — but for a good reason. He remembered his stint as a 'real' doctor, and how time-consuming it had been to fill out those infectious-disease forms that had to be fed into the government apparatus. Nowadays that was all done digitally. But it was still an unnecessary burden on doctors and nurses.

They already had their hands full with the flaming forest.

The East Asian way

On Tuesday 5 May, the chief magician of the United Kingdom was forced to resign. The day before, *The Daily Telegraph* had uncovered an affair Neil Ferguson had been having with a married 38-year-old woman for several weeks.

In typical, no-holds-barred British newspaper fashion, almost everything about the relationship was reported: the woman was living in an open relationship with her husband. And Ferguson himself did not live, as he said, in a 'traditional relationship' with his wife.

But it wasn't because of his alleged adultery that Ferguson was forced to leave his post as a government adviser, but because he'd broken the very restrictions he had helped to design.

During the UK's continuing lockdown, it was more or less illegal to leave your home. The only exceptions were for medical emergencies, daily exercise, food shopping, and certain types of work.

The police authorities in England and Wales had already fined 9,000 people for breaking the rules. According to *The Daily Telegraph*, that corresponded to one fine every five minutes.

Ferguson was far from the only legislator or decision-maker to break his own rules. The chief medical officer of Scotland had already been forced to resign after making several trips to her second home.

Before the pandemic was over, many a revealing article would be written about people who were happy to close down societies but had a harder time closing down their own lives.

But it was still early May. And in Sweden, news of Ferguson's exit was received with glee.

'This shows the absurdity of a lockdown. If he can't even follow the rules, how are others supposed to?' remarked one of the Swedish government's state secretaries.

The debate about closing down Sweden had long been over. Its strongest proponents had fallen silent.

From the rest of the world, more and more reports were coming in about ill health among young people increasing during their forced isolation. Two months had gone by since schools around the world had closed. Those who had hoped that digital solutions would prove a full and complete substitute for in-person teaching were forced to rethink.

No one wanted to close all Swedish schools anymore.

But at the same time, the Swedish death toll had begun to climb. The miserable weeks Denis Coulombier had warned of had been exactly that. Now almost 3,000 Swedes had died. If the Covid-19 pandemic was indeed to end up on a par with a serious flu, people had to stop dying — soon.

Every day at a 2.00 pm press conference, Anders Tegnell showed his diagram of the number of deaths. And every time, it looked pretty hopeful. It always seemed as though the number of daily deaths had peaked a couple of weeks earlier and was now dropping, slowly but steadily.

The diagrams were shared on social media across the world. For those who believed in the Swedish path, it looked as though the long-awaited herd immunity had kicked in and that Sweden would soon go back to normal.

But the reporting from Swedish hospitals was slow. Tegnell knew this. He usually reminded his listeners at the press conferences about the delay himself, but he was still beginning to hope that the number of deaths was on a downward trend.

From the Stockholm School of Economics, Adam Altmejd — like many other Swedes — followed the press conferences. He was a post-doctoral researcher in economics, and knew a thing or two about data visualisation.

He noted that Anders Tegnell seemed to believe that the delay only applied to the past week, when deaths were, in fact, being reported as far as three weeks back.

He's walking into his own trap, Altmejd thought.

So he wrote some code and put together his own chart. It contained both reported deaths and a prediction of how many additional deaths would be reported — if the delay remained consistent.

It offered a slightly different picture. The figures presented by the Public Health Agency on 3 May showed that 60 Swedes had died a week before that date — on Sunday 26 April. But in Altmejd's diagram, the corresponding figure should have been 77.

The actual number of deaths on that day would, much later, turn out to be 74.

Ironically, this delay meant that the 22 scientists who had published their infamous op-ed a few weeks previously would prove to be a little more right in hindsight.

The actual death toll on the days covered in the article — 7, 8, and 9 April — was now found to be 114, 96, and 106. This was 50 per cent higher than the Public Health Agency's claim that 60 to 65 people had died each day, was almost identical to the figure of 105 that had been cited by the 22 scientists, and was much higher than the numbers Tegnell had presented in his press conference that day.

Yet there were several reasons to believe that Sweden had seen the worst of the pandemic. The number of patients hospitalised in the country's intensive-care units was high, but it had stopped growing about a week before. The healthcare system's intensive-care capacity had been scaled up at breakneck speed. A field hospital had been erected in Älvsjö, south of Stockholm, but the 600 beds had not been needed.

And the number of new deaths had peaked at some point around mid-April. However, they remained on a plateau. More people were still dying in Sweden than in Norway, Denmark, and Finland put together.

And the awaited decline kept getting pushed further and further into the future.

Slowly, it began to dawn on the Swedes that this was no regular flu. But neither did they think it was the plague that the rest of the world believed it to be. Was there a middle way?

Now the spotlight began to be turned onto the tests. Ulf Kristersson wasn't the only one fascinated by the East Asian way. During the spring, technocrats around the world had proposed their own testing strategies.

For there had to be another way than Chinese-inspired lockdown politics.

One of them was the American Paul Romer. He had previously been chief economist at the World Bank, and was a notorious free thinker — the kind who gave TED talks and launched big ideas. His most famous idea was to build Hong Kong–like sanctuaries in Africa. Another time, he had suggested that Sweden should rent out its northern, less populated parts, and take in millions of refugees. Two years previously, in 2018, Romer had won the Nobel Prize in economics (the one that Swedes insist on calling 'the economics prize', as it isn't a 'real' Nobel Prize).

Like many other economists, Romer was of the opinion that the world's economies — indeed, the whole Western lifestyle — were being annihilated by the measures being taken to combat the virus.

So why not pour a fortune into building up a massive testing capacity? Next to all these other costs, it was cheap.

'The key to solving the financial crisis is to lessen the fear of getting sick if you go to work or go to a shop. It's about building confidence,' Romer explained.

Ulf Kristersson had the world's economic elite at his back. He had the head of the WHO on his side.

And finally, he got the government, too.

On 8 May, the minister for health and social affairs, Lena Hallengren, had no choice but to telephone the elephants' graveyard.

The elephants' graveyard was the mythical place in the Government Offices where former directors-general and other public managers ended up while awaiting new assignments.

Here, you'd find directors fired after some scandal, sacked county governors, managers whose agencies had been closed down, or people who had simply displeased the government in some way.

At the graveyard was Harriet Wallberg. She had been fired from her job as university chancellor in 2016 after Paolo Macchiarini, a scientist at the Karolinska Institute, had implanted artificial tracheas into eight patients, killing seven of them.

It was a scandal that shook the scientific world. Wallberg, in her role as head of the government supervisory authority, wasn't the only one who'd been let go. The entire board of the Karolinska Institute became collateral in the clean-up.

Now she was rehabilitated. On the morning of 8 May, a Friday, Lena Hallengren asked Wallberg if she wanted to take charge of those tests which, rather rapidly, had become such a hot political topic. Did she want to be the testing coordinator?

When do I start? Wallberg asked.

There's a press conference today, the minister replied.

Ulf Kristersson had hauled his idea all the way to the finish line.

There was only one problem. The purpose of the mass testing now being initiated across the world wasn't just to clamp down on the virus — the objective was also to reopen the economy. This was a problem that Sweden didn't have. Here, everything was already open. And Swedes were anything but scared of the virus. People crowded the shops, travelled to their summer houses, swam in public pools, and went to school.

The Swedish Covid hedonism had even become its own genre in the foreign media. Newspapers and TV channels around the world sent their reporters and photographers on safari in the brazen country.

For the citizens of its neighbouring countries, Sweden functioned as a release valve against the lockdowns. Norwegians went to their second homes in Sweden, while Danes travelled across the Öresund Bridge to get a haircut.

More extreme forms of Covid tourism were also reported. *Aftonbladet* wrote about rich Europeans flying into Stockholm to go to restaurants and nightclubs — pleasures they were denied in their home countries.

There was no doubt that Sweden's economy had many problems. Because the country's business model was basically to export forest products, trucks, and digital services abroad, it didn't matter much that 10 million Swedes were allowed to do as they pleased throughout the spring. This was a small country by the world's standards. The big companies were big because they had foreign customers. Now their foreign customers were sitting at home, watching Netflix.

Fear of the virus among the public wasn't one of Sweden's problems. But now the politicians had nevertheless decided that Swedes would be subjected to mass testing.

Sweden's politicians had taken their first step into the china shop.

Back to the drawing board

At the beginning of May, results were expected to roll in from those large-scale antibody studies.

At the Public Health Agency, hopes were that they would yield high figures. According to the agency's calculations, by 1 May around 26 per cent of the population in Stockholm County should have been infected with Covid-19.

Because the testing had been carried out just under a month before — at the beginning of April — the figures didn't have to be quite that high. The numbers now presented should show that at least 15 per cent of Stockholmers had antibodies.

The agency's mathematical model assumed that 17 per cent of the population in Stockholm should have been infected with the coronavirus a month before — on 11 April, to be specific. According to the same model, the peak — the day with the highest number of infectious individuals in the county — should have occurred on 8 April.

Tom Britton's — somewhat simpler — model came up with a similar prediction.

But when the initial results from the antibody studies came, they were both disheartening and unequivocal. Out of Niclas Roxhed's 1,000 envelopes, 550 had been returned. Of these, 446 tests had been correctly executed.

The results?

By mid-April, only one-tenth of Stockholmers carried antibodies against the new coronavirus.

Björn Olsen and Åke Lundkvist's testing of their friends and acquaintances showed similar results. Of the scientists' 453 friends and acquaintances of acquaintances, only 7.5 per cent had antibodies in their blood.

Even Torbjörn Sjöström's opinion poll pointed in the same direction.

At the time the tests were carried out, 9 per cent of Stockholmers believed they had been infected with the virus.

Other countries were seeing similar results. On 13 May, a study was presented showing that only 5 per cent of Spaniards were carrying antibodies — even though more than 25,000 had died of Covid-19.

But the Public Health Agency had its own study in the works. It had been a little delayed, but perhaps it would yield better results?

Pretty much every day, Anders Tegnell was asked when the study would be ready.

A week after the news from Spain was reported — on 20 May — the Swedish verdict came in: only 7.3 per cent of Stockholmers had antibodies. In the southern region of Skåne, the corresponding figure was 4.2 per cent, and in south-western Västra Götaland it was 3.7 per cent.

Regardless of who was doing the measuring — or how they did it — the results were remarkably similar. Very few people in hard-hit areas such as Madrid and Stockholm had antibodies.

Because the level required for herd immunity was assumed to be somewhere around 60 per cent, it seemed the pandemic could go on for a long time.

And by now more than 4,000 Swedes had died while carrying the virus.

For Jan Albert, the uncertainty had grown. Perhaps it would take longer for the country to reach herd immunity than they'd previously thought. At the same time, he had become increasingly certain that this wasn't the only variable that needed to be taken into account.

'The uncertainty is great, but we have to believe that we'll reach herd immunity. We can't keep societies closed down like this forever while we wait for a vaccine,' he was quoted as saying in *Svenska Dagbladet*.

There was no good alternative.

Only a percentage point or two had separated Tom Britton's prediction of the number of infections from the Public Health Agency's, but the difference between their reactions to the results of the antibody studies was more marked.

Anders Tegnell didn't budge an inch. To the country's journalists, he said the results corresponded to the Public Health Agency's models — but also that the patient group in their study hadn't been as representative as it ought to.

The agency would simply have to do a new study.

Britton was more shaken up. Had he made a mistake? Could the virus have been spreading faster than they thought at the beginning of the outbreak? Could there be people who'd been infected but didn't have antibodies?

He didn't tell him, but he thought Tegnell's reaction was strange.

Something had obviously gone wrong.

On the evening of 20 May, Britton went on Sweden's Television once again. The message he brought was a disheartening one: 'We'll have to go back to the drawing board.'

Tom Britton wasn't the only one who left the stage for a while. It was as though almost everyone in the drama took a little break towards the end of the spring, including that dissenting band of scientists — 'the 22' — who'd been taunted in so many columns and tweets that most of them had withdrawn from public life.

Then Johan Giesecke fell silent.

On 28 May, the journalist Emanuel Karlsten wrote on his blog that Giesecke had been on the Public Health Agency's payroll when he'd spoken in a range of TV shows and news articles as though he were an independent expert. This sparked a media storm that, in truth, was a bit peculiar. Anyone browsing the news archives could see that Giesecke had informed several media outlets — both Swedish and foreign ones — that he now worked for Anders Tegnell.

Those who had got to know him thought perhaps this was the first time in all of Johan Giesecke's life that he had been accused of *not saying enough*. After all, here was a man completely incapable of saying something he didn't think, and of thinking something he didn't say.

Careless and unguarded? Perhaps. Dishonest? No.

Nevertheless, a veritable shitstorm ensued. The Swedish strategy was now so hotly contested both in Sweden and abroad that every sliver of new information was used to attack the opposition's arguments.

Giesecke took it hard. He'd been a government employee almost all his life, but no one had ever requested his emails before.

He remembered something that his dad, the old rep of the powerful employers' association, had said: 'Don't spit your snus into the wind, and don't ever get into a fight with the media.'

So he laid low for a while, but he'd be back.

Then there was Anders Wallensten. His was a peculiar story. Most people in the virus business would have given their right hand to be deputy state epidemiologist at the height of the most notorious pandemic in a hundred years. But not Anders the younger. He went on leave to finish a book about diet, health, and exercise. It was a bit like being assistant manager of the national football team and taking your summer vacation the same month as the World Cup.

On 3 June, news came that Harriet Wallberg had quit. Her sojourn as national testing coordinator — or her leave from the elephants' graveyard, whichever way you chose to look at it — had lasted all of three weeks. What had happened was still shrouded in mystery. Wallberg herself claimed that the Public Health Agency's resistance to testing had made her job impossible.

Johan Giesecke's timeout lasted even shorter. The sixth of June was Sweden's National Day, and the old epidemiologist was invited to give a National Day speech in his home municipality of Södertälje.

He accepted. Now he was back.

What are you going to say, Anders Tegnell wanted to know.

Something patriotic, Giesecke replied.

And, just like that, summer had arrived.

Part V

The Swedish flu

The 1918 epidemic that came to be known as the Spanish flu did not get its name because it originated in Spain, or because Spain was hit exceptionally hard by the outbreak.

The name arose because, at the time, many countries were engaged in the First World War. Spain was neutral and had no wartime censorship. Its newspapers were thus allowed to write about the mysterious illness — so that's where people talked about it. By the time rumours of the contagion spread across the world, the name had stuck.

The role Sweden played in the Covid-19 pandemic resembled the one played by Spain during the Spanish flu quite a bit.

In the first few months the world was living with the new virus, thousands of studies were produced. Some were hopeful, others depressing. Sometimes the mortality figures were said to be low, sometimes high.

From Sweden came news of both kinds, but it was as though positive news found more fertile ground there.

Across the globe, the established media agreed that the world was facing an enormous threat. But in Sweden, that discussion was still alive. The debate raging in the country — about mortality figures, about the meaningfulness of restrictions — was unique.

So even though few of the affected countries censored their citizens — China being the biggest exception — it was as though the world's media kept having to turn to Sweden and its experts for a different perspective on the virus spreading across the world.

It wasn't just Johan Giesecke and Anders Tegnell who appeared on foreign TV channels and in newspapers. The paediatrician Jonas Ludvigsson was interviewed in several American papers about the importance of keeping schools open; Jan Albert told CNN that closing down society simply pushed the epidemic into the future; Tom Britton explained his models to *Forbes*, *The New York Times*, and others. The epidemiologist Carina King at the Karolinska Institute (who, it should be noted, was British and fairly sceptical of Sweden's strategy) told *Wired* that there was 'weak evidence on children transmitting to each other or adults within school settings'. The sociologist Karl Wennberg was called on to explain how the world's countries had emulated each other into lockdown.

It appeared that Swedish researchers didn't just offer a different view on the Swedish experiment, but a different view on the virus itself and the world's response to it.

For this reason, it wasn't entirely unexpected that it was a group of scientists from the Karolinska Institute — 29 of them, to be exact — who, in yet another unreviewed study, provided the world with a new take on the coronavirus in June.

It was also the answer to the question Tom Britton had asked himself after the discouraging antibody studies: could there be people who had been infected but who didn't have antibodies?

Was there something else protecting us?

The letter T

At the top of your torso is a small gland known in medical language as the thymus. Several animals have this same organ. And for a long time, those interested in this little gland were mostly chefs. Veal sweetbread in a cream sauce or pan-fried lamb sweetbread are just two ways of serving it. In humans, the thymus was long seen as a kind of counterpart to the appendix — a meaningless vestige.

But in the late 1950s, the British doctor Jacques Miller began to conduct some experiments. He surgically removed the glands of newborn mice, put them into adult mice, and proceeded to inject the latter with a liquid giving them leukaemia. Then he reversed the process, swapping out the newborn mice for slightly older ones — and so on. Each tiny variable was changed, until he came to a conclusion: mice with an underdeveloped thymus were unable to fight the cancer.

This gland was not unimportant.

It seemed as though he was on to something. He kept experimenting.

Miller's most important discovery happened by chance. In his little mouse workshop, there were some mice that served as the equivalent of cars stripped for spare parts. Miller had removed their thymus, but had no other plans for them.

Soon he noticed that these mice always got sick and died quickly. They appeared to lack the ability to fight even the most minor attack.

When Miller collected blood samples from the mice without a thymus, he noticed that they had a lot fewer of a certain type of cell, a type of white blood cell. Because they appeared to be connected to the thymus, he called them T cells.

By the time the 29 scientists at the Karolinska Institute began to explore the significance of T cells for the novel coronavirus, a lot had happened in the immunological sciences.

More than 50 years had passed.

By now, it had been established that T cells actually formed in the bone marrow before maturing in the thymus. We had also learnt that there were many types of T cells.

We'll stop there. For anyone interested in learning more, there is always medical school.

At any rate, T cells specialised in recognising virus-infected cells. And after recovery from a viral infection, the T cells' memory could provide a kind of immunity.

The problem was that measuring the immunity provided by T cells was much harder. Analyses could only be carried out in specialised laboratories.

During the spring, the 29 scientists at the Karolinska Institute had begun to test the blood of 200 Swedes. Some of them had been hospitalised; others had simply spent their February break in the hard-hit Alps. Many had mild or no symptoms of Covid-19 whatsoever.

It turned out that several of those who had experienced no symptoms still showed T cell immunity. They may not have had antibodies — but they were still 'immune'.

Of the people donating blood in the month of May, 30 per cent carried T cells specific to Covid-19.

That was a lot more than the antibody tests had indicated.

And the figure that everyone was seeking — the one that would show how close Sweden was to herd immunity — could now be adjusted upward significantly.

The study from Karolinska had a major international impact. It showed that the world was closer to the end of the pandemic than most people thought.

And at the same time as the Karolinska study allowed the number of people who were immune to be adjusted upward, a Swedish mathematician was nearing the finish line of his new project.

Herd immunity 2.0

In his red-brick tower with elm trees outside the window, Tom Britton was tinkering with some numbers.

He was back at the drawing board.

The gigantic whiteboard covering the western wall of his office was covered in equations in blue, red, and green. Little empty circles, solid circles, and circles intersected by a diagonal line each represented infected, immune, and recovered individuals.

'Do not worry about your difficulties in mathematics,' were the words on a poster covering the inside of the door. It showed an Albert Einstein lost in thought. 'I can assure you mine are still greater,' the cardigan-clad physicist told Britton and his students every day.

Sometimes Tom Britton fired off an email to Anders Tegnell or Johan Giesecke. Sometimes to an epidemiologist or mathematician out in the world. Sometimes he cycled over to the TV building at the end of Karlavägen to explain to the Swedish people how something worked.

But mostly he was busy with his new little project.

The point of the project was to calculate how many people would have to be infected with the coronavirus before herd immunity kicked in.

For anyone following the media coverage about the pandemic over the previous few months, it seemed like a peculiar question. Didn't we already know?

For those who had memorised the equation to calculate herd immunity, the question may have appeared even more odd. If the level required was $1-1/R_0$, and the value of R_0 lay somewhere between 2 and 3, the answer must be somewhere between $1-1/2$ and $1-1/3$. That is, somewhere between 0.5 and 0.67.

Around 60 per cent, in other words. You could almost do the maths in your head.

* * *

The classic herd-immunity model works well in some contexts. If you vaccinate a lot of children against the measles, you can assume that anyone getting the shot becomes immune; and as all children are called in by their local health centre at a specific age, immunity will be distributed in an even and predictable pattern.

But when it comes to a virus spreading through society, that model doesn't work quite as well. If a 55-year-old middle manager in the finance industry goes skiing in Italy, picks up the infection, and then returns home, it's not reasonable to assume that he'll spread the virus evenly to the rest of Swedish society.

After three days, he's more likely to have infected other middle managers in the finance industry than he is to have given it to a bunch of welders in some town up north.

And some incidents of transmission matter more than others. If a boy gives the virus to his big sister, it doesn't drive the epidemic to the same degree as if our middle manager happens to give it to a train conductor or someone else engaging with a myriad of people.

We could go on and on. The relationship between the abstractions of modelling and the complexity of the real world is a problem as old as science itself.

When epidemiologists want to illustrate the problem, they sometimes tell an obviously apocryphal story.

It's about some scientists who have achieved such a level of perfection in their work that the maps they draw keep getting bigger and bigger. Eventually, they draw a map that, when rolled out, covers the entire kingdom. The story has been retold in several ways by authors such as Lewis Carroll and Jorge Luis Borges, and pinpoints the difficulty in striking a balance between usefulness and precision.

Tom Britton worked on tiny maps. Compared to what other mathematicians and epidemiologists were doing, his models were small and easy to follow. With this new project, he took a tiny step towards the gigantic map. It wasn't a big leap, but it did mark a small increase in complexity.

Instead of assuming that the novel coronavirus would spread evenly across society, Britton attempted to build a model that assumed the virus would spread in different ways.

This was known as heterogeneous transmission. Neil Ferguson and Imperial College hadn't included such an assumption in their model, which was a little peculiar considering its complexity in other respects.

Britton sliced up the population a few different ways. The initial cuts divided up the Swedes by age. He chose six age groups, of which the oldest contained everyone over the age of 60.

Then he divided those into three different groups, based on how many people they interacted with: low activity, average activity, and high activity.

In the first group — those who mingled the least — you might imagine people in the countryside; adults with no children, perhaps; people who took the car to work, where they only had one or two colleagues; or individuals who, for other reasons, didn't run into a lot of new people in a regular day.

The most active group was easy to imagine. Here you had 27-year-olds who, on a regular Friday, would take the bus to work, grab lunch with their colleagues, and hit the gym in the afternoon before making an appearance at some house party in a crowded apartment.

In other words, people didn't all behave the same way.

Tom Britton already knew that each new layer of heterogeneity would lower the figure for herd immunity that the model spat back out.

It was pretty obvious when you thought about it. The people who see other people the most will be the first ones to become immune. And because these people — through their behaviour — have the biggest potential of spreading the infection, their immunity is 'worth more'.

There was another way of expressing this: removing a 27-year-old in Stockholm from the equation lowered the value of R_0 more than removing a forester in the far north.

When Britton was done, he assumed an R_0 of 2.5. In the classic herd-immunity model, an R_0 of that level would mean a herd-immunity threshold at 1-1/2.5 — that is, at 60 per cent of the population.

But his new, heterogeneous model produced a much lower figure: herd immunity would kick in when 40 to 45 per cent of Swedes had been infected.

If this was true, it was very good news for the Public Health Agency

— and for Tom Britton, who had increasingly come to be associated with the Swedish strategy.

And it wasn't just the threshold for herd immunity that could be lowered. If the study from the Karolinska Institute was correct, it meant that reaching the desired level of immunity was also much closer.

If 7 per cent carried antibodies, and 30 per cent had immunity from T cells, and herd immunity kicked in as early as at 40 to 45 per cent, there wasn't far to go.

Compared to the feeling of just a week or two before — when everyone thought Sweden had walked 7 miles down a 60-mile road — they now had only 5 or 6 miles left of a 45-mile journey.

Yet the perhaps most fascinating results came when Britton adjusted the model based on different levels of political measures to combat the virus — non-pharmaceutical interventions.

The varying degrees of severity of the restrictions were reminiscent of the scenarios used by Imperial College to illustrate the importance of drastic measures, which had subsequently sent several countries into extensive lockdowns.

Tom Britton chose four different levels — no measures at all, fairly small, fairly big, and very extensive — and assumed that all measures were introduced on the same day and, two months later, were lifted at the same time for a three-month period.

This is what people thought would happen at the time. Countries that had entered into a hard lockdown were expected to gradually reopen their societies over the summer months.

As one might expect, Britton's model showed that the measures would help delay the epidemic. Imposing some restrictions on movement in society was clearly a good idea. But in countries imposing the strictest measures, more people would eventually be infected than in countries taking the middle way.

The reason was that in hardline countries, the epidemic would have been quelled too soon. When society opened up again, there would be so many receptive individuals left that the epidemic could gain momentum once more.

On 23 June, Tom Britton's study was published in the journal *Science*.

* * *

Now two things had happened that, in one fell swoop, changed the preconditions for the unofficial part of the Swedish strategy: that a growing immunity would soon slow the spread of the virus.

First, the Swedish population had come closer to the finish line. If you believed the 29 scientists at the Karolinska Institute, antibodies weren't everything. To the portion of Swedes carrying detected antibodies, an unknown number of people with T cell immunity had to be added.

And the finish line had moved closer, too. Judging by Tom Britton's calculations, if a little over four out of every 10 Swedes became infected, that would be enough for the whole country to reach herd immunity.

Feeling optimistic involved several assumptions and unknown variables. But the most important number of all was both certain and hopeful. The number of people dying in Sweden had been falling for a long time, and was now down to fewer than 20 people per day.

Something had happened. But what?

Were fewer people dying because Swedes were good at keeping their distance? Or was it because they'd been so bad at it — thus building immunity? Or was it simply because of the warmer Swedish weather?

War rhetoric

Over the summer months, the results of the first Covid wave began to be tallied in the media.

There were different ways of measuring the devastation. One way of looking at it was that many people had died — more than half a million around the world by the end of June.

Another way of looking at the pandemic was that measures taken to combat it had frozen a lot of the functions in society that many exposed and vulnerable people struggled to be without.

For those who preferred the first perspective, there was plenty of data to lean on. Meticulous records of the death toll were being kept in most countries, especially the wealthy ones, and presented in stylish graphs on various sites: the Johns Hopkins University website, Worldometer, Our World in Data.

It was a lot harder to measure the consequences of the lockdowns. They appeared here and there as scattered anecdotes and figures. Perhaps the most striking data point came from the US: by the end of the school year, a total of 55.1 million students had been affected by school closures.

But, so far, the death toll was more interesting.

In early summer, *The New York Times* had published a front page completely devoid of pictures. Instead, it contained a long list of people who had died: a thousand names, followed by their age, location, and a very brief description.

'Alan Lund, 81, Washington, conductor with "the most amazing ear".'

'Harvey Bayard, 88, New York, grew up directly across the street from the old Yankee Stadium.'

And so on.

It was *The New York Times'* national editor who had noticed that the US death toll was about to pass 100,000, and so wanted to create something memorable, something you could look back on in a hundred years to understand what society was going through.

Those in charge of the paper's layout chose to draw up a front page reminiscent of what a newspaper might have looked like in the 1800s: a block of text without any big headlines.

The idea was for the names to become like a fabric of human lives.

The front page was reminiscent of what a newspaper might look like during a bloody war. It brought to mind the way American TV stations had reported the names of fallen soldiers at the end of every day during the Vietnam War.

The idea spread quickly across the world. A few weeks later, in Sweden, the front page of *Dagens Nyheter* was covered with 49 colour photographs below the words: 'One Day, 118 Lives'.

Those 118 people had passed away on 15 April. It was the highest daily death toll recorded throughout the spring. Since then, it had steadily been falling.

When Johan Giesecke read the paper, it left him a little puzzled.

On any normal day, 275 people die in Sweden, he thought.

He'd spent a large part of his life studying just that: where, when, and how people die.

The way the world currently thought about death was, to him, completely alien.

He'd taken part in an online conference in Johannesburg. One participant had pointed out that, that year alone, more than 2 million people had died of starvation in the world. During the same period, Covid-19 had claimed between 200,000 and 300,000 lives.

Giesecke felt as though the world was going through a self-inflicted global disaster. If things had simply been left to run their course, it would have been over by now.

Instead, millions of children were being deprived of their education. In some countries, they weren't even allowed to go to the playground. From Spain came stories of parents sneaking down into parking garages with their children to let them run around.

Tens of thousands of surgeries had been postponed by healthcare services. Screenings for everything from cervical to prostate cancer were put on ice.

This wasn't just happening in other countries. Sweden had seen its fair share of peculiar decisions, too. The Swedish police hadn't tested drivers for insobriety for months, in fear of the virus.

This year, it didn't seem quite as serious if someone were to get killed by a drunk driver.

It was becoming obvious that the media, the politicians, and the public had a hard time assessing the risks of the new virus. To most people, the figures didn't mean anything. But they saw the healthcare services getting overwhelmed in several countries. They heard the testimonies from nurses and doctors.

What the reporting didn't mention was that similar scenes had played out during the flu season of 2017–18. In both the US and Spain, hospitals had been forced to turn patients away, raise triage tents, and cancel planned operations.

When reporters wrote about it back then, it wasn't because people were dying, but because the problems shone a light on the strain on the healthcare system in several countries.

For a long time, hospitals' resources for events like these had periodically been boosted and cut. After the threat of bird flu, hospitals in the US had been given money to meet the demands of a future flu pandemic. But after the false alarm of the swine flu in 2009, the funds had dried up.

Here and there in the world — in Germany, the UK, Ecuador — people had been taking to the streets lately to protest the rules, laws, and decrees curtailing their lives. From other countries came reports that people were starting to flout the restrictions.

But the force of the resistance remained weaker than Giesecke had expected. There had been no French revolution, no global backlash.

One explanation for the citizens' passivity might have been the coverage of the deadliness of the virus in the media; it seemed they had been fed a non-contextualised picture of how serious the Covid-19 pandemic really was.

During the spring and summer, the global consultancy firm Kekst CNC had asked people in five big democracies — the UK, Germany, France, the US, and Japan — about all kinds of things relating to the virus and society. The sixth country in the survey was Sweden.

Sweden was a lot smaller than the other countries, but was included due to the unique path it was taking through the pandemic.

The questions were about everything, ranging from people's opinions on actions taken by the authorities, to the state of the job market, and on whether they thought their governments were providing sufficient support to trade and industry.

The twelfth and final topic in the survey contained two questions: 'How many people in your country have had the coronavirus? How many people in your country have died?'

At the same time as increasingly reliable figures were trickling in with regard to the actual deadliness of Covid-19, there was now a study of the number that people *believed* had died.

In the US, the average guess in mid-July was that 9 per cent of the population had died. If that had been true, it would have corresponded to almost 30 million Americans deaths.

The death toll was thus overestimated by 22,500 per cent — or 225 times over.

In the UK as well as in France and Sweden, the death toll was exaggerated a hundredfold. The Swedish guess of 6 per cent would have corresponded to 600,000 deaths in the country. By then, the official death toll was more than 5,000 and inching closer to 6,000.

Reporting the average guess was perhaps a little misrepresentative, as some people replied with very high numbers. In the UK, the most common answer was that around 1 per cent of the population had died — in other words, a lot less than the 7 per cent average.

But it was still a figure that overestimated the number of deaths more than tenfold. At this point, 44,000 Brits had been registered dead — or around 0.07 per cent of the population.

The breakdown of the numbers further showed that more than one-third of the Brits responded with a figure of over 5 per cent of the population.

This would have been like the whole population of Wales dropping dead. It would have meant many times more Brits dying of Covid-19 than during the entire Second World War — civilian and military casualties included.

The war rhetoric brandished by the leaders of the world had had an impact. Their citizens really did believe they were living through a war.

Face masks

Over the summer, the Public Health Agency began to space out its press conferences. In place of daily briefings, the press were invited on Tuesdays and Thursdays.

From the podium where Anders Tegnell gave his presentations, he could quickly spot the foreign journalists.

It wasn't because they were wearing other clothing, or because their hair looked different. It was because they wore a mouth covering.

Within the healthcare services, such pieces of fabric were known in Swedish as *munskydd* — roughly 'mouth covers'. But as people in other countries had begun to wear them, the word *ansiktsmask* — a direct translation of the English 'face mask'— crept into the Swedish language during the summer months.

It turned out that way because the Public Health Agency didn't want to talk much about those masks.

It led to some confusion at the big pharmacies. When people came in asking for 'face masks', they were shown to the skincare aisle, which displayed various facial treatments and creams for both ageing and dirty skin.

What struck Anders Tegnell from up there on the podium was that the journalists — they came from CBS, France1, the BBC, ZDF, and other foreign media outlets — clearly had no idea how to use their face masks. They were constantly poking themselves in the face, taking them off and putting them back on again.

Personally, Tegnell thought that wearing a face mask was unpleasant, and he had no intention of forcing Swedes to wear them. Even in the pandemic plan instituted in November 2019, he and the agency had determined that face masks had 'little effect' on transmission.

But in the rest of the world, the use of face masks was becoming more and more common. In countries that had closed down all activity, it turned into a kind of substitution therapy for their inhabitants. Their governments had been forcing the strongest drug imaginable down their throats for months, and now they were being given something a little more tolerable to put in — or over — their mouths. As though they were transitioning from heroin to Subutex.

In the UK, politicians even spoke of face masks as a means of getting people comfortable venturing back out into society. If they wore face masks, they could start going into shops and restart the paralysed economy.

Really, it was the same thing as with the mass testing initiated around the world. The purpose wasn't only to reduce transmission, but also to find a way for societies to open back up.

When the ECDC had wanted to recommend face masks in April, Anders Tegnell had sent them a critical email in return. He warned them against going public with the advice. He cited several different reasons, but fundamentally they all came down to the same thing: there was no scientific evidence to indicate that the use of face masks on a large scale was effective.

The arguments against using them were 'just as convincing', according to Tegnell. They could lead people not yet infected to take risks they otherwise wouldn't.

Besides, the 'communication' might suffer, as most countries had so far advised their populations not to wear face masks.

The advice published by the ECDC three days later was cautiously phrased. Face masks 'could be considered', it said, particularly in crowded spaces. But it also said that face masks should only serve as a complement to existing measures.

Yet, during the summer, the situation was becoming more acute.

On 22 July, the ECDC, together with the European Commission and the European Union Agency for Railways, began to recommend the wearing of face masks on train journeys.

Still, Anders Tegnell refused to follow suit.

In the same way as during the spring, when gyms and ski runs remained open in Sweden, several companies — those operating in multiple countries — were now faced with a choice. Should they follow the recommendations of EU agencies or the Swedish authorities?

Should they apply different rules in different countries?

Over a few decades, the Danish capital, Copenhagen, had gradually begun to merge with the Swedish city of Malmö, on the other side of the water. Trains shuttled unimpeded between the two countries across the Öresund Bridge, like any regular commuter train.

But starting in August, face masks were mandatory on all Danish trains — so when the train crossed the border from east to west, travellers had to get their masks out of their pockets.

The background to the confusion stemmed — as did so much else that year — from differing interpretations of the science, and not least Anders Tegnell's high demands of the scientific evidence.

At the beginning of the summer, *The Lancet* had published a study about the effectiveness of face masks and social distancing. Those advocating mandatory masking could pick out a few sentences here and there; analyses indicated that face masks had a protective effect — particularly among healthcare workers. Shielding one's eyes offered another layer of protection against infection. But the study also concluded that none of these interventions offered complete protection, and that optimal use required 'risk assessment and several contextual considerations'.

Keeping your distance was one thing: it worked, without a doubt. Recommendations about keeping at least one metre's distance led to a 'large reduction' in the number of infections.

Tegnell thought the study was done well — and that it showed the Swedish recommendations to be at the right level. Social distancing worked. Face masks, on the other hand, might even do more harm than good. He was supported by a medical commentary from *Läkartidningen*, in which the chief physician and professor Kjell Torén summed up the state of play in the research world: 'Weak Evidence for Face Masks Reducing Infection among the Public'.

But by this time, large parts of the scientific community had begun to think differently. Instead of demanding evidence, they demanded *caution*. In a critical comment to the news agency AFP, the epidemiologist K.K. Cheng at the University of Birmingham said that Tegnell's reasoning was 'irresponsible' and 'stubborn', calling on him to change course.

'If he's wrong, it costs life. If I'm wrong, what harm does it do?'

In several countries, face masks served as a political marker. In the US, many started taking pictures of themselves wearing a mask to use on social media. There were even apps being built that would make it possible to paste face masks onto existing images. Partly, some people used it as a way of distancing themselves from Donald Trump's views on the subject. The US president had expressed his scepticism of face masks on several occasions.

Many who were critical of the Public Health Agency's strategy now began to wear face masks on social media. One of them was Fredrik Elgh, who wore a big black mask on his Twitter profile.

But judging by most Swedes' behaviour, they agreed with their state epidemiologist about the dubious value of face masks. Wearing them wasn't prohibited but, so far, few could be seen doing it.

Not even when they were free were masks particularly popular. That summer, when the train operator MTR, the Hong Kong company, resolved its dilemma over all the different recommendations by distributing free masks to customers on its inter-city trains, it created an involuntary little experiment. About one in every three travellers grabbed a mask.

The trust in the Public Health Agency's recommendations was evident in other, more extensive surveys. In July, the proportion of the population that masked up was around five times greater in France and Germany than in Sweden.

There seemed to be a certain co-variation between the Swedish people's use of face masks and their attitude to the Public Health Agency's strategy. The just over 15 per cent of Swedes who at this time wore face masks while shopping or travelling on public transport — despite not being advised to do so — made up roughly the same proportion of the population who were negative about the agency's strategy. An extensive survey conducted by Gothenburg University would eventually show that, during the first summer of Covid-19, more than 80 per cent of the population had confidence in the Public Health Agency.

The Swedish people believed in their epidemiologists. This was clear to see, both in the opinion polls and on the streets.

Part VI

Tegnell's paradox

When autumn came, things were looking good for the people who were in one way or another responsible for Sweden's Covid strategy.

Throughout August, the death toll had remained low. Only a few Covid deaths per day had been reported. Moreover, most countries had reopened their schools. On this point, it did indeed seem as though Johan Giesecke had been right.

Anders Tegnell believed the rest of the world would now be hit harder by a second wave, and that Sweden would get off more lightly. With so many people already infected, he said, the level of immunity in Sweden should be high.

He didn't use the term 'herd immunity' anymore. But the thinking was basically the same. Sweden had allowed some transmission of the virus — while others had tried to stop it at all costs.

As the rest of the world now opened up more and more, one central tenet of the Swedish strategy would truly be put to the test.

The hopes of a presumedly high level of resistance — whether it came from antibodies, T cells, or herd-immunity threshold effects — weren't entirely unproblematic. Not many had paid it much attention, but during the spring Tegnell had sent out two conflicting messages.

On the one hand, he claimed that Sweden had managed to suppress the virus; this showed that their voluntary measures were working. On the other, he claimed that more people had had the infection than in other countries.

One of the people who pointed out the contradiction was the political scientist Anders Sundell of Gothenburg University. He called it 'Tegnell's paradox': *We don't want you to get the virus, but we want you to have had it.*

In one of the first books to be written about the pandemic, the American historian Peter Baldwin offered a critical interpretation of what the concept meant: 'In fact, the Swedish authorities did not trust their citizens to do the right thing. Their tactics presumed they would fail, in the process building up herd immunity.'

Things were a little more complicated than that. The experts' interest in how many Swedes had been infected, as we know, didn't solely have to do with immunity; it was also important information for determining how deadly — how dangerous — the virus was.

Considering how important the guesses of its mortality had been when the countries of the world closed down their societies, it was strange that there wasn't greater interest in calculating a truer figure. A few studies had popped up here, a few there, but there was no real agreement on how dangerous the virus really was.

According to the Public Health Agency's calculations for Stockholm County, the infection fatality rate was extremely dependent on the age of the infected. For those under 50, the fatality rate was only 0.01 per cent. For those over 70, however, it was 4.3 per cent. The proportion of the total population that had died from Covid-19 was estimated at 0.1 per cent.

According to official Swedish figures, almost 6,000 people had died. If 1 million Swedes had been infected, that meant the fatality rate was 0.6 per cent. If 2 million Swedes had been infected, that number was 0.3 per cent. And so on.

But now it was autumn. And, hopefully, the paradox no longer mattered.

Perhaps now Sweden could have its cake and eat it, too.

The responsibility for the high death toll was also beginning to be shared by more members across the community. A few months previously, the local paper *Eskilstuna-Kuriren* had revealed that the National Board of Health and Welfare had issued guidelines that caused several elderly people to be denied hospital care. This was a slow-burning story that would eventually explode when the journalist Maciej Zaremba wrote an article in *Dagens Nyheter* showing that Region Stockholm had dismissed particularly frail patients.

At the same time, the debate about the lack of testing at the start of the pandemic had degenerated into something reminiscent of a political science seminar. Did Sweden have too many regions? What did the division of responsibility between the regions, the authorities, and the government really look like?

During the summer, Johan Giesecke had largely checked out of Swedish public life. Now the pressure on Anders Tegnell began to ease up, too. And then, one Sunday in early autumn, the greatest proof of trust was bestowed on Tegnell since the start of the pandemic.

Downing Street

On the evening of 20 September, Anders Tegnell tuned in to a video call that would eventually be of great significance for the course of events in the home country of epidemiology.

As the clock struck six in London, and seven in Linköping, Boris Johnson suddenly appeared on the Swede's screen. The British prime minister was sitting at the end of the convexly shaped mahogany table around which the British government typically gathered.

Now there were only two of them at the table. Sitting next to Johnson was a 40-year-old man whose well-pruned side-parting and thick black hair revealed that he went to the hairdresser a lot more often than his boss did. The man's name was Rishi Sunak, and he was the chancellor of the exchequer. He was the one behind the little video conference now taking place.

Throughout the summer and the beginning of autumn, the spread of the virus had slowly but steadily been on the rise in the UK. There was now a big fear that the National Health Service would be struck by chaos as autumn turned to winter. Boris Johnson's scientific adviser had fixed on a solution they were calling a 'circuit-breaker lockdown'. The idea was to suppress the virus through a short and focused shutdown of society, thus creating a little breathing room. Simply put, the idea was to cut the power for a while — before turning it back on again.

Like the other lockdowns in the world, like the mass testing now being carried out in the US, Asia, and Europe, and like the contact-tracing apps launched in several countries, this was a form of newly invented social engineering. No one knew if it was going to work.

Rishi Sunak did not like the idea. The spring lockdown had pulverised the British economy. During the first quarter of the year, the country's GDP had fallen by 2 per cent. And through April, May, and June, it had fallen by another 18 per cent.

Sweden had fared a lot better. During the first quarter, its economy even grew a little. During the second quarter, it did shrink by 8 per cent, but that was better than the EU average — and a lot better than in the UK.

While others worried about the virus spreading, Rishi Sunak worried about unemployment. His figures showed that half a million Brits were at risk of losing their jobs that autumn.

Anders Tegnell wasn't the only one who had been invited for a digital visit to the British government's conference room. Also on Johnson and Sunak's screen that night were Sunetra Gupta — the Oxford scientist who'd done battle with those from Imperial College — as well as the doctor and epidemiologist Carl Heneghan.

Heneghan, too, was from Oxford. He was head of the university's Centre for Evidence-Based Medicine, and had long been trying to make the British government change its tough policies in favour of a more 'Swedish' line. Often, he'd broadcast his thoughts through his column in *The Spectator*, but this was his opportunity to influence the prime minister directly.

Alongside the trio of lockdown sceptics — Gupta, Heneghan, and Tegnell — a fourth scientist had been invited. He was John Edmunds, professor at the London School of Hygiene and Tropical Medicine.

Early in the epidemic, in March, Edmunds had advocated a herd-immunity strategy, and had even debated the subject with Tomas Pueyo on British television. Now, however, he stood behind the group of government advisers wanting to flick the switch for a while.

They each had 15 minutes of speaking time. Anders Tegnell delivered his usual shtick — the one he'd refined in thousands of interviews — about restrictions needing to be sustainable over time, and how reducing transmission on a voluntary basis worked just as well as legislation and government decrees. He avoided speaking about herd immunity.

The three lockdown-sceptical academics agreed that another lockdown was unnecessary. If society's most vulnerable members could be protected, lighter restrictions would suffice.

Tegnell and Gupta had rather similar thoughts about the pandemic. Both of them viewed it from a wider public-health perspective than did many of the advisers the British government otherwise relied on.

But if Tegnell's reason was that this was because he was following his agency's appropriation directions, for Gupta it was more personal. She viewed society from a leftist perspective, and was passionately critical of how school closures and ruined job opportunities during the spring lockdown had hit the least well-off in society.

Allowing airborne viruses to become endemic — that is, permanent and seasonal — was part of the social contract, she argued. When decision-makers clamped down on the spread of the coronavirus at all costs, it upset the balance in society. She argued that the British people — in fact, most people around the world except for the Swedes — had become stuck on one side of Aristotle's triangle of rhetoric (consisting of 'ethos', 'logos', and 'pathos', for anyone struggling to remember philosophy class).

The worldwide arguments now being cited in support of extensive lockdowns had emotional and moral overtones. The final corner — 'logos', the one referring to reason and evidence — had been forgotten. The world was out of balance.

Sunetra Gupta had hoped a lively discussion would ensue between the scientists, the Swedish state epidemiologist, and the politicians, but this did not happen. Johnson and Sunak listened, asked targeted questions, and noted down the answers without delving deeper into the issues.

Nevertheless, the meeting still had the effect that Sunak had been hoping for. Boris Johnson, who had seemed convinced about the value of closing down two days previously, now chose to wait.

Everyone involved promised not to mention anything about the meeting afterward.

It was as though things came full circle for Anders Tegnell that evening. Almost six months ago to the day, he had — both privately and in public settings — praised the British strategy.

Then he'd had to go it alone, like some coloniser on one of the empire's forgotten islands in the middle of the ocean.

And now he was advising the prime minister of the United Kingdom.

Perhaps it wasn't so strange that Johnson and Sunak asked him to keep the meeting secret. In British public life, Sweden and Tegnell had taken on all but mythical status.

Few noted the fact that the Swedish death toll — both in absolute numbers and per capita — was lower than the British. The prevailing image of Tegnell and his agency — in the UK, as in other countries — was that they had killed 6,000 Swedes. Perhaps not in cold blood, but at least with some kind of wilful neglect.

If it really was the case that so many people had died of Covid. Because now Anders Tegnell had a new question.

What had the Swedes *actually* died of?

Dry tinder

On 30 September 1839, Edwin Chadwick wrote an angry letter to the registrar-general of the United Kingdom. Chadwick was the secretary of the Poor Law Commission — the agency charged with easing the burden on the poor in England and Wales.

He had his work cut out for him. Over roughly half a century, the Industrial Revolution had driven a large part of the British population into factories that were hazardous to their health. Cities grew, overcrowding was on the rise, new technologies opened up for child labour, and conditions of production created widespread poverty.

Mortality was high. But what were impoverished people dying of?

This was the question addressed in Edwin Chadwick's letter.

Chadwick was a proponent of 'the sanitary idea', which suggested it was the filthy water, poor toilets, and resulting infections that killed people. In other words, people were dying of *diseases*.

In his letter, Chadwick complained about what one of the agency's employees was up to. The name of the employee was William Farr. He had grown up in poverty, but by the age of seven he had been offered an apprenticeship with a rich family friend. Eventually, he had trained as a doctor.

But the area in which he showed real talent turned out to be statistics. This was the reason he was now working as an unknown bureaucrat at the government agency in charge of recording births, marriages, and deaths in the country. Two years previously, in 1837, the Brits had begun to gather and analyse the causes of people's deaths.

This was during the infancy of modern medical statistics. And it wasn't obvious what type of information should be gathered, or even what to do with it.

What Chadwick complained about in his letter was an analysis conducted by William Farr of 148,000 reported deaths. Of these, Farr was saying, 63 people had died of *starvation*.

What's more, Farr had written that the actual starvation figure was even higher, but that the effects of hunger manifested themselves 'indirectly, in the production of diseases of various kinds'.

His conclusion bugged Chadwick for several reasons. In part, because it criticised his own work; in part, because Chadwick wanted to bring the nation's statisticians to focus on the diseases that were the direct cause of death — not on the underlying factors.

The correspondence that ensued between the two men was illustrative of the dilemma faced by medicine, epidemiology, and public-health statistics.

What were people *actually* dying of?

Edwin Chadwick held a position that was modern at the time. His approach anticipated the germ theory that would become so influential in the second half of the nineteenth century.

Over the decades that followed, Ignaz Semmelweis would advise his fellow doctors to wash their hands, Louis Pasteur would discover that heating milk ever so slightly made it safe to drink, and Robert Koch would isolate the bacteria causing anthrax and tuberculosis — all based on the revolutionary insight that diseases were caused by tiny, invisible microorganisms.

William Farr's approach was more traditional.

In the minds of a previous generation of doctors, typhus wasn't caused by a bacterium — but by hunger. For them, epidemics weren't so much a symptom of a disease moving through a population as indicators of the amount of suffering in that population: of poverty, overcrowding, excessively hard labour, nutrient-poor foods, and everything else slowly but surely wearing down the human body.

A disease taking over a human body was like a spark igniting a dried-out tree trunk.

The spark was just what lit the flame. But the dryness was the real reason it caught on fire.

William Farr's thinking would sometimes lead him astray. When London was hit by several cholera outbreaks in the mid-nineteenth century, he investigated the issue thoroughly. Across more than 300 pages, full of maps and tables, he discussed a number of factors that could explain how and why some people were affected: the patient's age, sex, the amount of rain in the area, property prices, wind directions, population density.

But the vast amount of data turned into an obstacle, rather than an asset.

The conclusion Farr finally settled on was that the disease had topographical causes. The higher up you lived, the lower the risk that you'd get sick with cholera.

His observation wasn't completely silly. To this day, some scientists study the impact of elevation above bodies of water during cholera outbreaks in poorer countries. But Farr's theory wasn't correct.

Instead, it was the doctor John Snow who solved the mystery. By marking out all the deaths on a map, he could see that many of them were concentrated around a single water pump in the city.

Samples from the pump showed the water to be completely clear, however, so Snow decided that small quantities of an infection were enough to get sick.

John Snow died four years later, at the mere age of 45, in the aftermath of a stroke. But by the time London was hit by yet another outbreak in 1866, Farr had accepted Snow's theory that cholera was a waterborne disease. He was one of few doctors in the city to believe in it at the time.

Farr collected water samples, and discovered that one of the companies supplying water to London was using a reservoir that had long been discarded due to contamination.

Paradoxically, William Farr thus became the man who ensured that John Snow's ideas lived on.

Even though William Farr's thinking belonged to an older tradition, there was something modern about his way of reasoning. Today, what we call science is often focused on analysing complex processes by looking at a number of underlying factors. When crime goes up or down in a society, its cause can be traced to everything from political reforms to demographic changes and technological developments. When a person falls sick with a serious illness, the cause is often a combination of genetics, upbringing, and behaviours.

Few things have only one cause.

William Farr would later go down as one of the big names in medical history — a bit like Sweden's own Carl Linnaeus.

Farr's classification of diseases laid the foundation for the International Statistical Classification of Diseases and Related Health Problems — or ICD — a system that is used all over the world today. For instance, Farr's legacy can be seen in the way some countries allow for *poverty* to be categorised as a cause of death.

And a century and a half later, his legacy manifested itself when a Swedish state epidemiologist began to ponder why so many Swedes had died.

Now it was September 2020 in Sweden. Things still looked calm. The number of reported deaths hovered around two to three per day.

By now, several countries had managed to surpass Sweden in the number of deaths per capita, but it remained high on the list. Number 12, to be exact.

Anders Tegnell had had time to think. Why was it that so many had died in Sweden? Or: what had the 6,000 Swedish victims of Covid *actually* died of?

The theory he formulated was like a carbon copy of William Farr's notion that mortality didn't just depend on the spark — but also on the dryness of the fuel.

Based on statistics compiled by the European public health agency, the ECDC, Tegnell had been able to determine that the annual influenza epidemic had hit both Norway and Finland harder than Sweden during the months before the coronavirus reached the Nordic countries.

Sweden — like the UK, Belgium, and the Netherlands — had had several years of low flu mortality. And the flu that had spread during the winter of 2019–20 had been exceptionally mild in Sweden.

In several interviews with various media outlets in mid-September, Tegnell formulated what would become known as his 'flu theory'.

In support of his theory, he also cited a study by three economists at the American Institute for Economic Research.

The study listed 15 possible explanations for why Sweden had been hit harder than its neighbouring countries. Among the possible reasons were the timing of the February school break in Stockholm; a certain lack of personal protective equipment across the regions; the high proportion of immigrants in the country; its large nursing homes; and the size of Stockholm compared to Oslo, Helsinki, or Copenhagen.

But the single most important explanation was Sweden's 'dry tinder'. According to the authors, fragility among the elderly could explain between 25 and 50 per cent of Sweden's deaths.

Once Anders Tegnell had presented his flu theory, the backlash came fast. Joacim Rocklöv argued that the differences in deaths weren't significant enough to serve as an explanation. From Finland, Mika Salminen said Tegnell was half-right: there had admittedly been 'more frail old people' in Sweden than in Finland at the start of the year, but that was only part of the explanation.

In Norway, Frode Forland was more critical. The main reason why so many had died, he argued, was that more of the elderly had been infected in Sweden.

It had been 161 years — almost to the day — since Edwin Chadwick had written his letter to William Farr's boss. And now, Anders Tegnell was arguing with Frode Forland, Joacim Rocklöv, and his other critics about the exact same thing.

Had 6,000 Swedes died of *a disease* or of *frailty*?

The control group

It wasn't so strange that the issue of the Swedish death toll was engaging so many people outside Sweden's borders. When scientists conduct experiments, there is a concept known as 'placebo controls'. When a new drug is tested, half of all participants are given the real medication while the other half are given an ineffective sugar pill. The latter is referred to as the control group.

The idea is that comparing the two groups will allow you to study whether the drug has been effective.

Six months previously, the countries of the world had initiated a large-scale experiment by closing down their societies.

And the Swedes became the control group.

But that's not how the situation had been described in countries under lockdown. In the eyes of the foreign media, Sweden was the country that had initiated a painful human experiment.

The Guardian likened the strategy to a game of Russian roulette, calling it 'deadly folly', while the German magazine *Focus* equated the policy with 'sloppiness', and the Italian *La Repubblica* wrote that 'the Nordic model country' was making a dangerous mistake.

One of the agencies under the Swedish Ministry for Foreign Affairs conducted a survey showing that interest in Sweden had never been this high among the traditional media. It forced foreign minister Annika Linde to call a meeting with the diplomats the country had sent out into the world. Her message was to focus on correcting the image of Sweden. It wasn't at all the case that Swedes were ignoring the virus. The voluntary measures were just as effective — perhaps even more effective — in preventing the spread. Swedes were not some death-defying hedonists.

The effort hadn't been particularly effective. The world's media continued to be fascinated by what was now known as 'the Swedish experiment'.

And finally, one day in July, *The New York Times* itself — the US 'paper of record' — chronicled Sweden's fall from model country to deterring example: 'Sweden Tries Out a New Status: Pariah State'.

The country's unofficial foreign minister — Johan Giesecke — wasn't perturbed. He remained wholly convinced that Sweden had chosen the right path through the pandemic.

Johan Giesecke had won lots of small victories lately. He had climbed another rung in the complicated hierarchy of the WHO and was now the vice chair of its Strategic and Technical Advisory Group for Infectious Hazards. He had also convinced the group to get behind a letter he'd sent to the director-general of the WHO, with the message that lockdown was an inappropriate strategy for poorer countries.

It was a bad idea that had spread across the world: from China to the West to Africa. In poorer countries, lockdowns caused even more problems than in richer ones: vaccinations ceased, so did girls' education, and workers living hand to mouth were quickly left destitute.

Three days after Anders Tegnell had his meeting with Boris Johnson, Johan Giesecke was invited to advise politicians in Ireland.

On Wednesday 23 September, he once again peered through the camera hole on his MacBook from his study at Skärfsta Gård. Far away, on the other side of the North Sea, the old epidemiologist's face was blown up on a large TV screen mounted in a conference room in Oireachtas, the Irish parliament.

Giesecke started by explaining that he'd in no way been sent to represent Sweden.

'I used to work for Sweden. But I'm now just Johan Giesecke,' he began.

The people seated in the room over in Ireland were members of its parliamentary Covid-19 committee. And what they heard that day was an unfettered Giesecke, freed from all political considerations and from all those wary officials who had been toning down his message for so long.

A few weeks before, his contract with the Public Health Agency had been terminated. Now he was simply — and fully — Johan Giesecke.

He explained Sweden's strategy. And he thought Ireland should copy it.

'You should allow controlled spread of the disease for people below sixty.'

There was no need for any 'policing in the street'.

'People are not stupid. If you tell them what they should do to protect themselves and others, they will generally follow what you tell them.'

It was true, he said, that the poor and marginalised were hit hardest by the virus. But they were also hit hardest by the restrictions.

Such was the testimony from the control group in Scandinavia.

The Irish should take the sugar pill.

The ideas about herd immunity were one thing. As yet, it was hard to assess whether the Swedish people carried any significant immunity. As yet, no one knew whether countries that had closed down would now be hit hard — or whether Sweden would experience a second wave.

But there was another component of the Swedish strategy that became subject to increasing debate.

The Swedes were still free.

During the spring, the French had been forced to jot down on paper what errands they needed to run before leaving their homes. Now — as the virus spread across the South American continent — Argentinian children had to sneak into closed playgrounds. In several countries, people of faith were not allowed to attend public worship. Political parties were not allowed to meet. In Germany, demonstrations were declared illegal. A dusk-to-dawn curfew had been imposed in several countries.

This wasn't just a fight between Daniel Bernoulli and d'Alembert — about what risks to expose a population to. Not just a struggle between William Farr and Edwin Chadwick — about causes of death. It was also a revival of Thomas Hobbes versus John Locke — a debate older than modern democracy, about the appropriate balance between liberty and security in society.

This was the philosophical question that Benjamin Franklin once answered with his famous words that a society willing to give up a little freedom to gain a little safety deserves neither — and will lose both.

Perhaps it wasn't so strange that it was neoliberal and conservative-minded people, primarily in the US, who rejoiced in the Swedish trust in individuals to make their own choice. Perhaps, they wrote, Sweden had listened to the advice given to the politicians of the world by the economics prize winner Friedrich Hayek in his 1974 Nobel lecture in Stockholm? Perhaps they had listened when he said: 'Act humbly with your great powers.'

But it was — as so much else during the 2020 pandemic year — a little more complicated than that.

Science!

Sweden's new status — as an outpost of liberty or as a country conducting a death-defying experiment, depending on who you asked — wasn't solely the result of the choice it had made when it had come to an epidemiological crossroads. It also had to do with the country getting caught up in a much wider political conflict.

That conflict — as so much else — was centred in the US.

Back in the day, decades ago, the education level of American voters wasn't particularly decisive in predicting which party they'd choose. But in recent elections, voters with high educational attainment had increasingly been drawn to the Democrats, while those who hadn't gone to college were drawn to the Republicans.

Among political scientists, this phenomenon was known as 'the diploma divide'.

During the 2016 presidential election, this divide grew even wider. It was particularly pronounced among white voters: of those without a college degree, 67 per cent voted for Donald Trump.

Trump's surprising win was seen by some as part of a wider populist movement sweeping across the West. A few months previously, the Brits had voted to leave the EU, and populist parties were making strides in most of Europe.

After the US election, *The New York Times* put up billboards with the word 'Truth' in metre-high letters. The message was that our fact-driven, scientific-minded society, a precondition for democracy, was under threat from the new administration settling into the White House. 'Truth. It's more important now than ever,' read the full ad.

Donald Trump undoubtedly had a special attitude to facts. According to a breakdown by *The Washington Post*, in his first three years in office Trump managed to make 16,241 false or misleading claims.

In the rest of the world, it was primarily the Trump administration's stance on global warming that drew attention. Despite the scientific consensus that greenhouse-gas emissions pose a threat to the societies of the world, the new administration chose to scrap environmental laws, even withdrawing from the Paris Agreement.

Ahead of the 2020 spring, a large part of the American public saw their government as anti-scientific. At the same time, Trump's popularity was interpreted as a revolt by the other half of the population against experts, against the elites wanting to run every detail of their lives.

The same impulses existed in the UK. 'The people of this country have had enough of experts,' the powerful conservative politician and then justice secretary Michael Gove had said ahead of the Brexit referendum in 2016.

It wasn't just *The New York Times* that sided with the experts and knowledge society. Traditional media outlets all over Europe were fighting the populist wave. At the beginning of February, Donald Trump began to comment on the novel coronavirus. He said it would go away in a month or so, that the warm weather would help, and that one day, 'like a miracle', it would disappear.

In the UK, Prime Minister Boris Johnson was initially just as dismissive. Tirelessly, he continued to shake people's hands and skipped several meetings about the new virus.

During the spring and summer, Donald Trump stayed the course. He said that 99 per cent of cases were 'totally harmless' and that children were practically immune.

At the same time, the US Centers for Disease Control and Prevention, the CDC, made a very different assessment — as did a well-known member of the president's own pandemic 'task force'. The doctor and immunologist Anthony Fauci had become renowned in the US during the AIDS epidemic 40 years earlier. As early as 1981, he'd begun to research possible treatments for the unknown HIV virus, but due to the authorities' botched handling of the epidemic he was long blamed for the country's failures. Eventually, however, his image in the media changed — and Fauci was declared something of a hero. Over the coming decades, he would travel around the world and accept awards from various scientific academies. He was awarded the National Medal of Science by George W. Bush; Barack Obama hung the Presidential Medal of Freedom around his neck.

In March 2020, the decorated scientist — by then 79 — made the assessment that the new coronavirus was ten times deadlier than a regular flu. He thereby joined the ranks of those who advocated tough measures to combat its spread. That month, a voluntary quarantine and other federal guidelines were also introduced.

The problem was that Donald Trump, like many others around him, wanted to go in the other direction. The lockdowns in certain parts of the country — which were largely introduced at a state level — had already caused the economy to freeze.

This led to a tug of war within the government. By the end of March, Anthony Fauci, at any rate, managed to persuade the president to extend the federal guidelines for another month.

But on 13 April, the president retweeted a tweet from the Republican politician DeAnna Lorraine. It contained criticism of Fauci and ended with '#FireFauci'.

The next day, the hashtag was shared on Twitter by tens of thousands of users. And the media began to speculate whether Trump was about to fire the famous doctor from his task force.

Spokespersons for the White House denied it. And Trump himself professed his appreciation of Fauci.

But it was obvious there was a conflict between the experts and the politicians.

The US media boiled the dispute down to Fauci versus Trump. In this way, the fight was made part of the wider conflict between populism and expertise that had dominated Trump's first three years in office. Reinforcing that image was the fact that the states introducing the toughest and earliest closures — such as New York, New Jersey, and California — were governed by Democrats. States under Republican rule — including Georgia and Florida — chose a different path.

Fairly soon, a picture began to spread that Republican governors were ignoring scientists, and prioritising the economy. Democratic governors, on the other hand, listened to the experts, and protected lives.

On 4 May, the California governor, Gavin Newsom, tweeted that his state was 'led by data and SCIENCE' — with the word 'science' in all caps.

There were several details complicating that picture. Among other things, the early lockdowns in New York, New Jersey, and Massachusetts had to do with these states having been hit particularly hard by the virus. Their large, densely populated cities — with their highly educated, urban populations — were an underlying cause both of the high rate of transmission and of the Democrats' electoral victories there.

There were legal differences, too. Florida's constitution meant that important decisions were decentralised; it was largely up to those who governed the state's 67 counties to decide on certain measures.

But this was rarely discussed on TV networks and social-media channels, and in the newspapers, podcasts, and radio shows describing what was happening in the US. The fight over the virus turned into yet another battle in the war over the role of science in society.

Across the Atlantic, Johan Giesecke now found himself in a somewhat unexpected position. His own stance seemed suspiciously similar to Donald Trump's.

Would the pandemic soon be over? Yes.

Were most cases harmless? This was true.

Did children spread the virus? No.

Were the measures to combat the virus worse than the virus itself? Absolutely.

Many of the opinions he and the Public Health Agency held about the virus were deemed so dangerous by Facebook and Twitter that they were either removed or marked with warning flags when spoken by Donald Trump.

In a video posted to the president's Facebook and Twitter pages, Trump said that children were 'almost immune'.

'My view is the schools should open. This thing is going away. It will go away like things go away. And my view is that schools should be open,' the president said.

A few hours later, the video was removed by Facebook, which said in a statement that it violated the company's misinformation policy.

Soon after, Twitter followed suit. The explanation was the same as the one offered by Facebook. Trump's statement went against the company's rules on Covid-19 misinformation.

The next day, the Swedish immunologist and doctor Agnes Wold —

who was generally positive toward the Public Health Agency — wrote on Twitter that 'children don't fall sick when exposed to the virus. So called natural immunity, most likely.'

Yet her post was allowed to remain.

These were strange times. What was regarded as a scientific discussion in Sweden was deemed to be misinformation in other countries.

A meeting in Massachusetts

Two weeks after the video conference with Anders Tegnell and Boris Johnson, Sunetra Gupta travelled across the Atlantic, to a small town in the far west of the US state of Massachusetts. There, she met up with another Swede. His name was Martin Kulldorff. He was the one who had invited Gupta to the little town of Great Barrington.

Kulldorff was a statistician, epidemiologist, and professor of medicine at Harvard. During his career, he had authored articles with titles such as 'An Elliptic Spatial Scan Statistic' and 'Power Comparisons for Disease Clustering Tests'. They were as well-cited as they were impenetrable to lay readers, but during the pandemic he had started to become known outside his field of study as the author of op-eds in both Swedish and foreign papers. A few months earlier, he had even been awarded an honorary doctorate by the university in his hometown, Umeå.

Kulldorff wasn't just critical of lockdowns, but also of mass-testing the population. According to him, hunting asymptomatic infections only led to more lockdowns, and testing children only led to more missed schooldays.

Martin Kulldorff had nothing to do with the Swedish strategy. He had never met Anders Tegnell, and the two of them had only exchanged a few words via email throughout the year.

But in the US, Kulldorff had become a bit of an ambassador for the Swedish way.

A couple of weeks before, he'd advised Florida's governor, Ron DeSantis, in an online roundtable. He and the two Stanford scientists Jay Bhattacharya and Michael Levitt had been invited. Levitt was the 72-year-old Nobel Prize winner who had proposed his theories of saturation — the effect that arose when enough people had died of the virus. Bhattacharya was a professor of medicine, but had also been active within the field of economics. He had published scientific articles on everything from Russian alcohol mortality to links between health-insurance plans and obesity. Early in the pandemic, in April, he had taken part in conducting a famed antibody study in Santa Clara County, California, which showed that Covid-19 was less deadly than most people believed at the time.

Their conversation with Florida's governor lasted more than three hours — and, according to transcripts, the word 'Sweden' came up 21 times.

Kulldorff wasn't the only one who had talked about his home country. All four participants spoke of the little nation.

Sweden had kept its schools open. Sweden had trusted people's judgement. Sweden had a lower death toll per capita than the UK, Spain, the US, and several other countries that had closed down. And so on.

They weren't many, those scientists who questioned the world's lockdowns. But at least they'd found each other.

Like an endangered species, they had now gathered in a single herd. And far away in northern Europe was a nature reserve.

On 4 October, three of them — Bhattacharya, Kulldorff, and Gupta — gathered in Great Barrington to compose the herd's manifesto. The reason they ended up in Great Barrington, of all places, was that it was home to the American Institute for Economic Research, AIER.

The AIER was a libertarian think tank that had been advocating free-market solutions to social problems since 1933. During the pandemic, it had taken a stand against the lockdown policies of several countries. Moreover, the AIER had published the study offering 15 explanations for Sweden's death toll — the one that Anders Tegnell had referred to.

For a self-declared socialist such as Sunetra Gupta, the AIER was a strange bedfellow. But lockdown critics were few and far between; you had to make friends where you could. Besides, she saw value in the fact that their resistance didn't come from one political direction.

'Coming from both the left and right, and around the world, we have devoted our careers to protecting people. Current lockdown policies are producing devastating effects on short- and long-term public health.'

Fewer cancer screenings, lower vaccination rates for children in several countries, and deteriorating mental health were just a few of the consequences.

Aside from their explicit mention of herd immunity as something desirable, it was like a slightly more eloquent version of the Swedish strategy.

They named their manifesto 'The Great Barrington Declaration'.

Two ominous emails

At the same time as the meeting in Great Barrington was being held, two ominous emails popped up in Anders Tegnell's inbox.

Ever since the summer, Swedish society had gone into a kind of reflective mode. When the newspapers wrote about the Covid-19 pandemic, they'd quite often use verb forms signifying the past tense. Why hadn't Sweden engaged in contact tracing? How come so many patients in retirement homes hadn't been allowed to see a doctor? What happened with that contact-tracing app some government agency was supposed to build? Had Swedish legislation been inadequate for the situation the country had gone through?

Anders Tegnell was still convinced the pandemic would now hit the lockdown countries hard. When they could no longer bear to keep their societies closed, the virus would sweep in over France, Germany, Denmark, and Eastern Europe. Maybe even South Korea.

Sweden, on the other hand, had built up a certain immunity.

In a document sent to Sweden's administrative regions, different scenarios were outlined for what the autumn and following year might look like. The most likely outcome, according to Tegnell, was a low-grade transmission during the autumn, with a risk of local outbreaks in different parts of the country.

In other words, things were looking up.

But on 4 October, the scientist Marcus Buggert sent a long email addressed to both Tegnell and the head of the Public Health Agency's department for microbiology, Karin Tegmark Wisell.

Buggert was an assistant professor at the Karolinska Institute and one of the 29 scientists conducting the much-discussed study on T cells published a few months prior.

'The reason I'm writing this email,' he wrote, 'is that it has come to my attention that you are using our article, and perhaps also further calculations of which I may not be aware, to argue that more people have been infected with SARS-CoV-2 than antibody tests are indicating.'

Buggert explained that he was the article's corresponding author. This meant that he was the contact person for any queries having to do with the text or its contents.

'Personally, I find some writings about our results to be blown out of proportion and there to be nothing in our article that suggests we are closer to herd immunity or similar because of our results. The leap from our results to politics is way too big.'

The Public Health Agency wasn't the only body that had used the study. During the summer, it had found its way into the US Congress and become the subject of a question that the Republican doctor and congressman Mark Green had put to Anthony Fauci.

Fauci, too, had read the study from the Karolinska Institute — from 'the Swedes', as he called the 29 scientists. But in the congressional hearing, he held up another study, from the La Jolla Institute for Immunology, showing that many people with T cells had carried them since before the pandemic even began.

'This is work that we really need to pursue,' Fauci said. 'We're just at the cusp of understanding the importance of this type of response in Covid-19.'

Buggert's message to Tegnell and Tegmark Wisell was similar to that which Fauci had relayed to Mark Green: this research was still in its cradle.

In his email, Buggert tried to convey how complex the issue was. As he and his colleague had written in their article, between 20 and 50 per cent of the population had carried some level of T-cell protection even before the pandemic broke out — probably due to their previous exposure to another coronavirus.

Such T cells likely protected against severe Covid; but, unlike antibodies, they didn't offer *sterile* immunity. This meant they could still pass the virus on to others.

'I would just like to share my thoughts as I have become significantly more humble with regard to our results; especially as they have been used in too many scenarios as political incitements to open up societies in the US, UK, and other parts.'

Finally, he asked Tegnell and Tegmark Wisell not to use the article as an argument to prove that the virus was more widespread than indicated by antibody testing.

It ended up being Tegmark Wisell who wrote back to Buggert: 'Based on what you write below, we will be extra careful not to refer to your study in relation to any assumptions about the proportion not detected with antibodies but potentially with T-cell methodology.'

The next day, on 5 October at 10.00 in the evening, Tegnell received another email. The subject line read 'Quick uptick in Covid in Uppsala!'.

The sender was Johan Nöjd, an infectious-disease doctor in Uppsala. He wrote that they had identified 207 cases over the last seven-day period. This was more than double the number recorded the week before.

The virus appeared to be spreading across all age groups. Even more 'worryfully', Nöjd wrote, hospitalisations had skyrocketed. From having around five hospitalised patients for several weeks, they'd now gone to having 24.

Nöjd wrote that he needed help with testing. But what else should they do? Was there a signalling value in closing restaurants after 10.00 or 11.00 pm? Recommending face masks on crowded buses, perhaps? On commuter trains?

He signed off: 'Speak soon.'

Anders Tegnell wasn't quite ready to accept the thought that Sweden was about to be hit by a second wave.

During press conferences in October, he showed diagrams of the spread in other European countries instead. He thought the figures were dramatic. In the Netherlands, Denmark, and France, the curve was now beginning to shoot straight up. Even Germany seemed to be hit harder.

He wasn't the only one to notice that one of the hypotheses underpinning the Swedish strategy now appeared to be confirmed. In several of the countries now being hit by the second wave that Tegnell had predicted, journalists began to ask an uncomfortable question: 'Were we wrong about herd immunity?', as the Danish newspaper *Politiken* had mused a few weeks earlier.

The rapid surge in fascination for the Swedish strategy soon created a backlash. On 14 October, *The Lancet* published an open letter by 80 scientists from epidemiology, infectious medicine, and related disciplines.

They wrote that the renewed interest in a herd-immunity approach was 'a dangerous fallacy'. There was, they wrote, no evidence that undergoing the infection gave any lasting immunity. A herd-immunity strategy would only lead to recurring epidemics.

They called their open letter the 'John Snow Memorandum', after the doctor who had solved the mystery of cholera.

Great Barrington or John Snow? A Swedish strategy or a German-French-Spanish-Californian one? Just like in the spring, the battlelines were being drawn.

And just like in the spring, Sweden began to chart its own path through the coming autumn.

On 22 October, the government announced that the rules for public gatherings and official events would change. From 1 November, the limit for a seated audience would be raised from 50 to 300 people.

Throughout autumn, a number of debaters and members of the cultural sector had demanded an easing of the restrictions on their activities. Several times, the government had been asked why cultural and sporting events were curtailed by strict rules, while stores and shopping centres weren't.

For many, this was long-awaited news. But it was also a decision whose timing was bad.

The draught horse

Some of the individuals referring to themselves as infectious-disease doctors would say they weren't quite like other doctors.

One thing uniting many of them was that they weren't only interested in people. Considering that they worked on viruses and bacteria — which jumped between pigs, chickens, and people, and back again — it wasn't so strange that they would happily slice open a pig every now and then to see what was inside.

Among the famous infectious-disease specialists in the world, many cultivated an interest in other life forms. They were bird watchers and shepherds. They were fascinated by Guinea worms. They could offer a detailed account of how the black and white stripes of the zebra protected the animal against the tsetse fly.

Back in the day, when they first went to university, many of them had chosen between medicine and courses in biology, zoology, or veterinary medicine. If you listened closely, you could hear it when they spoke. Their language was full of zoological similes based on a knowledge of animals and biology such as few possessed.

'An Ardennes,' Björn Olsen said now. 'The virus is a bit like an Ardennes horse.'

There weren't many Ardennes horses left in Sweden — they had been used in agriculture before the time of the tractor. The Ardennes was calm and strong — not fast.

Björn Olsen was known for his mild, somewhat genteel, manner. He didn't like to speak badly of others. Even now — as he'd been drawn into the most acrimonious scientific debate in a generation — he couldn't keep himself from describing Anders Tegnell as 'knowledgeable' and Johan Giesecke as 'the grand old man of Swedish epidemiology'.

But, in truth, he thought both Tegnell and Giesecke were completely wrong about the way the virus spread. Another way of describing its slow, steady, almost patient expansion was that the virus spread in clusters: it penetrated a small group and blew up within it. Slowly and patiently, it appeared to be moving through the country's population — from one group to the next.

During the summer, the US infectious-disease agency, the CDC, had reconstructed the process through which a church choir in the state of Washington had been infected. Sixty-one people had been singing and having coffee together for a couple of hours. One of the choir members carried the virus, which was enough to infect 53 others. Three of them ended up in hospital, and two died.

The significance of this type of super-spreader event could explain why some countries and cities were hit hard, while others appeared to be faring better.

But despite most people agreeing on how the virus spread across the world, the information could be interpreted in different ways.

The interpretation expressed in the Public Health Agency's forecasts was that smaller — manageable — outbreaks here and there were now more likely.

Another interpretation was that the slowness of the virus made it possible to control its spread. If the virus wasn't sweeping indiscriminately through the population, intensive contact tracing, isolation, and strict lockdowns might actually work.

Like Johan Giesecke, Björn Olsen could quote Axel Oxenstierna, too: 'Carefully weigh, boldly decide, thus abide.' This was a sentence that Annika Linde, the previous state epidemiologist, had liked to quote. Olsen thought it summed up the attitude of Swedish bureaucrats pretty well.

And carefully weighing and boldly deciding were fine. But he didn't agree with the third part at all. You always had to re-examine your decisions. Especially concerning new viruses. There was so much you didn't know, and so much new information all the time.

Changing one's mind, he believed, was one of the virtues of the profession. After all, the viruses and bacteria were so many — and the infectious-disease doctors so few. They simply had to share information, listen to each other's theories — solve the mysteries together. Ever since the spring, Björn Olsen had believed there wouldn't be a second wave. Now he'd changed his mind.

Now he was sure it was coming.

The second wave

The rising numbers of reported cases of the virus sweeping across large parts of the European continent in the autumn were beginning to be referred to in the media as a 'second wave'.

Exactly what the term meant wasn't entirely clear. For some, a second wave implied that the virus had mutated and become more dangerous — which happened during the Spanish flu — while for others it simply meant that the first wave had yielded only low immunity in the population and that the disease was taking the opportunity to gain ground once more.

During the summer, the term had begun to be used in yet another way — in this case, to describe the rekindled spread of the virus in North America.

In the charts showing the number of cases in the US, it had looked like the country was already suffering another peak during the summer months. But what really happened was that the virus had begun to spread in states previously spared, such as Texas, Arizona, Alabama, and Louisiana.

Something similar was now beginning to happen in Sweden. Already by November, Region Skåne, which had only been very mildly affected in the spring, had more hospitalised Covid patients in inpatient care than ever before.

It was in part due to this terminological confusion that Anders Tegnell avoided calling the growing number of cases in Sweden a 'second wave' throughout most of November; it created too many associations with the way the flu usually behaved. And by now they knew this virus didn't behave like a regular flu.

In the diagrams summing up the situation in Sweden in various ways, it now looked as though something was starting to happen: the number of positive tests, the *proportion* of tests that came back positive, the number of hospitalisations — it was all on the rise.

But was it a second wave? Or was it a large number of new, smaller outbreaks, which in the aggregate looked like another wave?

After being badgered by journalists at a couple of press conferences, Anders Tegnell finally caved in and started referring to what was happening in Sweden as a second wave.

The second wave — if that's what it was — came to have big consequences for the Swedish strategy.

After all, this was exactly what wasn't supposed to happen. The Swedish population was supposed to be more protected this time around. Their built-up immunity was supposed to prevent yet another onslaught on the healthcare services.

It didn't take long for the effects to show in the Swedes' trust in their decision-makers. The proportion of Swedes who had a high level of confidence in the Public Health Agency now began to plummet — from 68 per cent in October to 52 per cent in December, according to the polling company Ipsos. The confidence in Tegnell would follow the same curve: from 72 to 59 per cent.

Immediately, the media scrutiny got stricter. The questions at the press conferences turned more critical. Tegnell's previous statements that Sweden wouldn't be hit by a second wave were picked apart in retrospect.

What wasn't clear in the media coverage during these weeks was that Tegnell's basic assumptions had largely turned out to be true: there appeared to be a protective immunity in the population. It was simply unevenly distributed across the country. Though the numbers of Covid-19 hospitalisations in intensive-care units were beginning to surpass spring levels in several parts of the country, things were looking better in others.

Stockholm offered the clearest example. Not once during the autumn and the coming winter would the number of intensive-care hospitalisations rise to more than half as many as during the spring. And of the total number of patients in the country's intensive-care units in November, Covid-19 patients only made up a fifth.

But such nuances were lost.

And now things were starting to happen fast.

The party's over

When the government finally decided to dismantle the Public Health Agency's strategy, things happened quickly — very quickly.

They started with the booze.

Throughout autumn, pictures and videos had been posted on social media of crowded dance floors, primarily from Stockholm's nightclub district around Stureplan.

Anders Tegnell hadn't expressed any particular concern when asked about the partying. But both Stefan Löfven and Mikael Damberg had announced their dismay.

'The partying will have to stop,' the prime minister said.

'It's deeply irresponsible and disrespectful,' said the minister for home affairs.

This was an optical issue; it didn't look good. Not when the media was reporting on a second wave. Not when the Allsvenskan football league was being forced to play without an audience. Not when gigantic, airy churches were only allowed to have 50 people at their services.

The nightclubs had to close. If not for reasons of infectious-disease control, then for political ones. But how? During a few months in the spring, there had been a temporary pandemic law that could be used, but it had expired in the summer.

Now the lawyers at the Government Offices showed an impressive creativity. They started by looking into a law about temporary infectious-disease-control measures in places serving food or drink. It gave the government powers to decide how these establishments should be organised, and how their premises should be designed, in order to prevent transmission. But the most effective measure would be to introduce a ban on selling alcohol. If that were done, who would be out late at night?

In the lawyers' assessment, the law did not allow the government to limit alcohol sales. So they kept looking. Finally, they found a regulation dating from 18 June 1937. It stated that alcoholic beverages could be prohibited 'in case of war, the immediate threat of war, unemployment, or a large-scale emergency or other extraordinary circumstances'.

That was it. On 11 November, the Ministry of Health and Social Affairs sent out their memorandum about a new regulation. Now, all alcohol sales — with a few obvious exceptions, including hotel minibars — would be prohibited after 10.00 pm.

A few days later — on 16 November — the prime minister stood in front of two Swedish flags, explaining that it would be prohibited to organise public gatherings and events with more than eight participants.

'Unfortunately, the coronavirus takes no heed of our feelings. For this reason, there is now a need for more bans to push down the curve of infections.'

Compared to measures introduced in other countries, these restrictions were fairly mild. Europe wasn't just undergoing a new wave of disease but a new wave of lockdowns, too.

Yet these new initiatives were remarkable for one more reason: this was the first time the government had so clearly chosen to override the Public Health Agency. Neither the ban on alcohol nor the so-called rule of eight were ideas the agency endorsed.

It was evident that if the government wanted to, it could.

Paradoxically, Sweden began to abandon the Swedish strategy around the same time that many of the predictions of its architects started to come true.

Much of what Johan Giesecke had predicted in the spring was now happening.

Several of the countries that had clamped down hard on the virus in the spring were no longer able to keep it at bay.

The US, France, Switzerland, Croatia, Mexico, Brazil, the Czech Republic, Slovenia, Argentina — the number of countries whose deaths per capita surpassed Sweden's kept on growing.

They were large and small. Rich and poor. And they were spread across the world.

Even Hungary — where 'the dark forces', as Giesecke liked to call them, were at their strongest, and where Viktor Orbán had invoked the threat of the virus to strengthen his power — now had more deaths per capita than Sweden.

On lists showing what proportion of the population had died in Europe, Sweden came in somewhere around the middle.

In the US, more than half of all states had been hit harder than Sweden. And now Germany began to catch up, too. During most of December, the death toll per capita there was higher than in Sweden.

Yet perhaps the most interesting case was the UK — the country that had shared the same strategy as Sweden for a few days, but then chosen to change tack. Despite a resolute lockdown during the spring — so powerful that it snuffed out a large part of the British economy — and a test-and-trace program for which the bill would eventually rise to £22 billion, by the end of December its total death toll per capita was 30 per cent higher than Sweden's.

But by this time, the politicians and experts of the world were so deeply mired in the lockdown paradigm that it didn't cross their minds to re-examine their hypotheses.

And then — at the end of the year — another weapon fell into the hands of the Covid warriors.

V-Day

Early in the morning of 8 December 2020, Margaret Keenan took a seat in a gigantic blue armchair at University Hospital Coventry in the UK. She was 90 years old, about to turn 91, and peeking out from under her unbuttoned grey cardigan was a blue T-shirt. Its print, soon to be famous, showed a penguin in a scarf and a Christmas hat.

A nurse walked up, asked whether she consented, and proceeded to stick a small needle into Keenan's left upper arm. It contained a vaccine called Comirnaty, developed by the companies Pfizer and BioNTech.

And just like that, Margaret Keenan became famous as the first person in the world to be vaccinated against the novel coronavirus.

It was a truth needing some modification. Tens of thousands had already been vaccinated in studies conducted around the world. AstraZeneca, Novartis, Johnson & Johnson, Sanofi, GlaxoSmithKline — pretty much all the big pharmaceutical companies had produced vaccine candidates. And they weren't the only ones: universities, start-ups, small drug companies — a considerable part of the medical world had been hard at work since the spring.

Enormous sums of money had been poured into the research. And it wasn't the companies' shareholders who were primarily taking the risk. In the UK alone, by December the government had already spent £12 billion on everything from research grants to orders of potential vaccines, according to the National Audit Office.

In the US, $18 billion had been set aside for what was known as Operation Warp Speed. The term 'warp speed' had been borrowed from the world of science fiction, and was perhaps best known from the TV series *Star Trek*. Travelling at warp speed meant to move at a velocity faster than the speed of light.

Of all the assumptions and predictions made by the Swedish Covid architects during the spring — once the virus had entered the country

— this was the only one that ended up being completely off the mark.

Both Anders Tegnell and Johan Giesecke had guessed that finding a vaccine would take years. Chances were, they believed, the pandemic would more or less be over before there was a cure.

They hadn't been alone in that assessment. As recently as in the summer, Pascal Soriot himself — the CEO of AstraZeneca — had said to the British paper *The Times* that during the pandemic the pharmaceutical companies were working against the clock.

The time constraint wasn't about bringing an end to the pandemic with a vaccine, but about pharmaceutical companies needing to test their vaccines before the worst of the spread was over.

For this reason, the WHO had published guidelines for so-called challenge trials — studies in which young people were intentionally infected to measure the efficacy of the vaccines.

But the virus hadn't subsided. And the pharmaceutical companies could gather enough data by natural means.

The absence of a vaccine was one of the central assumptions forming the basis for Sweden's chosen path: the longer it took to produce, the more unlikely it seemed that the world's societies would be able to hold out under extensive lockdowns.

Not putting their hopes in a vaccine was also one of the clear points of advice that Johan Giesecke had given the world's countries.

Yet now the vaccine was here.

It had happened very quickly. Already, by early November, results from vaccine trials by three different companies — Pfizer/BioNTech, Moderna, and AstraZeneca — had indicated strong protective effects.

The positive results had stirred the world's financial markets to life. Shares in companies selling cinema tickets, trips, hotel stays — things that had been frozen by the pandemic — began to rise rapidly. It was one of many signs that the world was starting to hope might mean things would soon go back to normal.

The blue penguin T-shirt worn by Margaret Keenan sold out in the Coventry hospital's online shop. More T-shirts were ordered in. They sold out, too.

The whole world was overcome with a fit of joy.

But the vaccines now quickly being approved by the world's

pharmaceutical agencies also had another, less noted effect.

Now lockdown advocates gained fresh oxygen. For if a vaccine was on the way, we might as well keep the lockdowns going a little longer, right?

The Covid generals of the world could dust off their war metaphors once more.

'The cavalry is coming,' Anthony Fauci exclaimed.

The UK health secretary, Matt Hancock, followed suit. He declared Tuesday 8 November 'V-Day' — 'V' for 'vaccination', in a reference to D-Day, when the Allied powers landed in Normandy during the Second World War.

This was a war that would go on far into the following year.

Mission creep

Johan Giesecke had taken his last swim of the year in Lake Uttran.

It was as it always is.

His wife lived by another principle. She kept on swimming until the lake froze.

And so, every morning throughout November, Giesecke would walk up onto their large balcony and anxiously follow his wife's movements until she was back on land. Then he'd head down to his office and start his workday.

If it was a Tuesday, he would dial in to his group at the WHO. Any other day, he'd have a chat with some old colleague, sometimes Anders Tegnell, perhaps a journalist in some faraway country.

It was a changed Johan Giesecke who sat there speaking. It was most obvious when he answered questions. Now, those replies that used to require no time to think were held back a few seconds.

This was what it was like to be a professor in a field of study that in the space of six months had leapt decades into the future.

In just half a year, the scientific discipline to which Giesecke had dedicated his life had undergone a metamorphosis. Now, measures that until a year ago had been completely unthinkable for stopping a respiratory tract infection had become *comme il faut*. The terminology had collapsed.

He knew he had made some miscalculations. The vaccine had arrived sooner than he'd expected. And he realised now that the virus spread differently than he'd thought. He, who had assumed that it would spread like an influenza — quickly, mercilessly, and impossible to stop — now realised this wasn't some tidal wave engulfing the world.

But it was fairly typical of the autumn of 2020 that tiny details concerning the properties of the virus were elevated, scrutinised, and discussed at length in the media.

Exactly how did the virus spread? How common was it for symptoms to linger long after an infection? Which face masks worked best? Were *two* masks better than one?

As the world zoomed in on the details, it lost interest in the bigger question, the immense uncertainty that had been a major reason why certain countries had chosen to go into lockdown.

The question of how dangerous the virus was. How deadly it actually was.

By now they knew much more. A review in the WHO's own *Bulletin of the World Health Organization* — building on 61 other studies — had shown that the median infection fatality rate was 0.27 per cent, but that it varied considerably between nations. The differences had to do with a number of factors: the age distribution in society, varying ways of counting deaths, and other things.

Bad as it was, this wasn't a new Spanish flu. It was no contagious variant of HIV. It wasn't close to the 3.2 per cent fatality rate — albeit a case fatality rate — that the WHO had reported during the spring and that had spread in the world's media.

'The inferred infection fatality rates tended to be much lower than estimates made earlier in the pandemic,' the study noted.

Johan Giesecke's early forecasts about the novel coronavirus being as deadly as a regular flu virus had been on the low side. Covid was worse, yet perhaps comparable to a severe flu, the kind that hit the world every decade or two.

He thought people had been spooked. And the fact that young people in some countries were still isolating, now that it was clear they ran a low risk of being severely affected, that was just silly.

During the early months of the pandemic, most people had agreed on the purpose of the measures imposed. In all countries, it pretty much came down to two things: avoiding unnecessary deaths and protecting healthcare services from an onslaught. Based on these goals, the decision-makers of the world chose to go with different measures — everything from mild recommendations to hard lockdowns.

But during the course of the year, something had happened. Slowly, new goals had crept into the politicians' rhetoric: reducing the number of cases, preventing people from getting sick, even bringing the number of Covid cases to zero. The latter strategy had been dubbed 'zero Covid' and was now being promoted by many of those who had wanted to shut down the world's societies early on: New Zealand's prime minister Jacinda Ardern; the 'hammer and the dance' originator, Tomas Pueyo; and in Sweden, among others, Björn Olsen.

If the fight against Covid was a war — as so many of the world's leaders proclaimed — this was the equivalent of what was known in armed conflicts as 'mission creep'.

The phenomenon had been observed on several occasions: a country went to war to achieve a certain goal, but as time passed that goal changed. When the US started sending troops to Vietnam in the 1960s, it was with the purpose of training the South Vietnamese army; a decade later, the country found itself immersed in a jungle war impossible to win. When the Iraq War started, it was initially justified with the goal of removing weapons of mass destruction from the country; when none were found, the rhetoric shifted to introducing democracy.

To many scientists around the world, these new demands for a total and unconditional capitulation were no doubt unrealistic. As we know, humanity had only ever been able to declare itself victorious over a virus once before. And the novel coronavirus had little in common with the smallpox virus, eradicated a few decades earlier.

When the journal *Nature* asked 100 virologists, immunologists, and infectious-disease researchers about the plans, most of them said it was an impossible pursuit. It was, as one American epidemiologist said, like 'trying to plan the construction of a stepping-stone pathway to the Moon'.

An insight began to grow that the virus was likely to become endemic — permanently existing in society — and that this was something we'd have to live with.

But the war against the novel coronavirus had long been a political project — not a medical one. And as of yet, there was nothing to indicate that the governments of the world felt like laying down their weapons.

The Irish politicians had not heeded Giesecke's advice. By now, the little island had imposed some of the toughest interventions in Europe.

And in Sweden, restrictions continued to tighten. Week by week.

Now Giesecke's country was going mad, too.

* * *

Finally, when only two weeks of the year remained, the death knell came for Sweden's chosen path through the pandemic.

In the beginning of summer, the government had, after pressure from the opposition, appointed a 'Corona Commission' to evaluate measures taken throughout the pandemic by the government, its agencies, the administrative regions, and the municipalities.

On 15 December, the commission presented the first in a series of reports. In the very first sentence of the press release that was circulated, the strategy to protect the elderly was declared to have failed.

By the time of the report's publication, more than 3,000 people in the country's nursing homes, and nearly 1,700 people with in-home care, had died of Covid-19.

Its 300 pages covered a lot — perhaps everything — of what was wrong with Swedish elder care; these were structural issues, known since long before the pandemic broke out. According to the report, there was also a lack of national oversight of the municipalities' preparedness.

But there was one sentence in the report — or, rather, in the press release — that stood out. It read: 'The general transmission in the community is likely the single most important factor behind the significant transmission in nursing homes.'

These were words with political power. They were picked up by opponents of the Swedish strategy, and quickly interpreted as saying that the mild measures were the main reason for the high Swedish death toll. *Dagens Nyheter*'s editor-in-chief, Peter Wolodarski — who had wanted to 'close down Sweden to protect Sweden' — wrote on Twitter that it was a 'key sentence'. In parliament, it was cited by critical members. The words were pasted into editorials in papers all over the country. The leader of the Christian Democrats, Ebba Busch, who'd said in a debate on Sweden's Television that 'Sweden had allowed large-scale transmission with deliberate malice' — something she'd been criticised harshly for — saw her reputation restored. It wasn't possible to protect at-risk groups, she said, while also having a high level of community transmission.

* * *

The report itself contained a lot more complexity. And when one of the commission's members, the Karolinska Institute professor Mats Thorslund, was asked by Sweden's Television whether there had been 'unnecessary deaths', he said it was too soon to tell.

But it wasn't surprising that this wording held explosive power. Around this time, the general consensus was that Sweden had been hit exceptionally hard during the pandemic — both from a historical perspective and compared to other countries. It was one of the presuppositions for the continuing public debate.

But it wasn't necessarily true.

Mortality and interpretation

One day in late 1993, a long-awaited play was about to premiere in Stockholm. Ingmar Bergman had directed the *Goldberg Variations* — a play by George Tabori promising to attack and question 'all old gods and conventional values' — and it was set to premiere on Saturday 11 December at the Royal Dramatic Theatre in Stockholm.

But a few days before the premiere, a small announcement appeared in one of the capital's papers. The show had been cancelled: one of the actors had come down with the flu.

Around the country, little messages now began to pop up — an announcement here, a news article there — about the workings of society getting interrupted by someone falling ill with the flu. The leader of the Left Party was forced to skip a debate about plans for a joint currency in Europe; three players in the national table tennis team dropped out of the semifinals in the European Championships League; and the musician Ola Magnell had to cancel a few shows.

The longer the winter wore on, the worse things got. Funeral directors noticed that they had more and more to do. Classrooms emptied. Hospitals filled up. Waiting times at children's emergency rooms grew longer and longer. Blood banks were drained when donors were unable to get to the hospital.

On 14 January, *Göteborgs-Posten*, the local paper in Sweden's second-largest city, reported that 37 bodies had been left on the floor of the Sahlgrenska Hospital because its morgue was full.

Two months later, *Expressen* wrote that, in a short time, one-fifth of all patients in a nursing home in Ljungbyhed had died. Those in charge of the home had offered to vaccinate everyone at a cost of 160 kronor each, but many felt that was too expensive.

In the article, the municipality's head of care stressed that they had followed all the rules. And perhaps old people dying wasn't so strange after all.

'Ten of the people who died were born before the Boer War,' he said. The paper renamed it the 'Death Home'.

The flu sweeping across the world in 1993–94 was one of the last to be given a geographical name. It was known as the Beijing flu, and it hit several countries hard. The reason was a mutation in the virus that meant that even those who had had a flu infection in preceding years lacked immunity.

Despite the high death toll, and despite the strain on the healthcare services, the Beijing virus quickly fell into collective oblivion. The way epidemics usually did.

But Anders Tegnell remembered it.

He had been 36 years old at the time, working as an infectious-disease doctor at Linköping University Hospital.

As he remembered it, patients lay strewn everywhere.

In 2020, the memory of the 1993 flu pandemic was brought to life again. This stemmed from the figures now being compiled of how many people had died in Sweden as the novel coronavirus spread through the population.

The death toll presented by the Public Health Agency at its press conferences and on its website each week was one thing: it was based on how many had passed away within 30 days of testing positive for Covid-19.

It had been the agency's decision to tally the numbers that way. But Anders Tegnell thought it was a poor indicator of how serious the epidemic was. Partly because countries had chosen different ways of counting their dead, partly because many who ended up in the Swedish statistics had died 'with Covid, not from Covid', as he liked to say.

On several occasions, people had come up with ideas for how he could present the figures differently. Johan Giesecke had tried as early as April to make him compare the Covid deaths to the regular, seasonal flu; outsiders had sent emails with other ideas.

They had received short replies from Tegnell, saying that he agreed, the way they were currently presenting the numbers was a problem, but they couldn't change it now.

So, several times a week, he got up in front of the TV cameras to explain how many deaths had been reported, based on an arbitrary definition he didn't really care for.

It was what everyone wanted to know. The figure everyone asked for. He couldn't do it any other way.

For more than a century — indeed, perhaps several centuries, if you recall John Graunt and his mortality tables — epidemiologists had preferred to measure the severity of epidemics in terms of the excess mortality they caused. That is, how many people had died compared to how many usually died.

One of the people who had been a driving force in developing this method of counting was William Farr — that British bureaucrat who insisted on searching for underlying factors for every death.

'The death rate is a fact,' he'd said. 'All else is inference.'

In May 2020, they had received their first piece of fact. That was when Statistics Sweden had revealed how many Swedes died in April.

It was a relevant month to study. By mid-April, preliminary deaths from Covid-19 had peaked. In a few days, more than 100 deaths had been recorded.

With the total fatality figures, it was now possible to assess how severe the epidemic had been. To make a historical comparison.

So, how many had died in total — of any cause — in April 2020?

The statisticians' answer: 10,458 Swedes had died.

That was a significant number of deaths. Very significant. It was the deadliest month in Sweden in almost 27 years — the deadliest since December 1993.

But what did it mean? Was it a disaster? A big crisis? A minor crisis? Nothing to worry about?

When Jan Albert read about the statistics, he sent the figures to Tom Britton and Anders Tegnell.

Tegnell thought they were interesting. Exciting, even. He wrote back to the mathematician and the doctor that he remembered 1993. That he'd been working in Linköping at the time. That there had been patients everywhere.

'But,' as he wrote to Albert and Britton, 'it wasn't a crisis.'

The prime minister goes shopping

On the morning of 19 December, a Saturday, Stefan Löfven and his wife were strolling along Regeringsgatan in Stockholm. It was just days before Christmas, and less than two weeks before the end of the turbulent year.

Ever since the beginning of March, Sweden's prime minister had managed to stay out of the limelight — all while some public servants, doctors, and epidemiologists ground each other down beyond recognition.

It was an astonishing political feat.

A year that had left such marks on the faces of Johan Giesecke, Anders Tegnell, Björn Olsen, and everyone else who'd somehow touched the Swedish strategy had left the head of government in a virginal state.

Anders Tegnell had been forced to find a secret location for his bike to keep it from getting vandalised outside Central Station. Johan Giesecke's private life and financial situation had been exposed in the press. Björn Olsen and Fredrik Elgh had been taunted on social media.

Anyone who had come into contact with the Swedish strategy in any way had been forced to pay a steep price.

But the prime minister had managed to remain surprisingly invisible.

It hadn't been easy. It had required a couple of well-timed speeches to the nation, and the appointment of a Covid-19 commission when things got heated.

It hadn't mattered hugely that, four days previously, this very commission — in its much-discussed interim report — had noted that 'the government rules the country' and thus also bore the ultimate responsibility for the transmission of the virus within elder care, the late introduction of a ban on visits to the country's nursing homes — indeed, everything that could explain the high death toll in Sweden. If it actually was significantly higher than in the rest of the world.

About this, those in the country proficient in arithmetic had, a little quietly, now begun to argue.

Most opinion polls, which had admittedly been conducted before the Covid commission published its first report, showed that confidence in the prime minister as well as support for the Social Democrats were back at about the same levels as before the virus began to spread on the European continent.

And now a vaccine was on the way. The year was almost over. Perhaps it wasn't so strange that Sweden's prime minister felt he could relax on that Saturday before Christmas, as he was walking down Regeringsgatan with his wife.

But then they stepped off the street.

The mistake Sweden's prime minister was now about to make was at once both surprising and inevitable.

Hundreds of politicians had already fallen into the same trap.

It started back in July, when New Zealand's minister of health was forced to resign after visiting a beach with his family, despite the 'level 4 lockdown' the country had imposed in the beginning of May. Shortly thereafter, it was Neil Ferguson — Professor Lockdown himself — meeting up with his mistress in London. In the summer, several of Ireland's top politicians had attended a golf banquet for 80 people — including the European commissioner for trade, Phil Hogan. In August, the Dutch minister of justice had hosted a big wedding.

And so it went: New York's mayor, Bill de Blasio; the mayor of Chicago, Lori Lightfoot; the Californian governor, Gavin Newsom; the US Speaker of the House, Nancy Pelosi; the former UK Labour leader Jeremy Corbyn; the British prime minister's adviser Dominic Cummings. The list went on and on and on.

The question was what conclusion to draw from the fact that the same individuals who had curtailed their people's liberties so often were caught breaking the very laws, restrictions, or recommendations they had introduced.

Was it aristocratic indifference?

Or was it simply proof that it was impossible to shut down your life — regardless of your social standing? That there was something deeply inhuman about the lockdowns the world had attempted during the year?

* * *

For most of 2020, Swedish politicians hadn't been forced to deal with that problem. The restrictions that had been introduced required active, intentional efforts to violate.

As long as the country's leaders didn't throw big parties or plan long-distance trips, they were safely within the bounds of the rules.

But the day before — on 18 December — Stefan Löfven had stood in front of the press and announced that indoor swimming pools, sports centres, and museums — places that were owned either by the municipality or by the state — would close. Selling alcohol after 8.00 pm was prohibited. The annual post-Christmas sale was off. Several times, the prime minister had stressed that Swedes should cancel all 'non-essential activities'.

A few days later, the City of Stockholm would begin to melt its outdoor ice rinks. A new pandemic law was coming. There had been one in the spring, but it had expired in the summer without ever being used.

From 10 January, pending approval by parliament, the government would have significantly greater powers to swiftly shut down various parts of society.

The media speculated that Sweden was finally headed towards a lockdown. It seemed as though the Swedish experiment had come to the end of the road.

Stefan Löfven and his wife turned right, and stepped inside the enormous shopping centre.

It was 10.00 am, and the shops had just opened.

The shopping centre was empty. Very empty. The people of Stockholm had heeded the new advice and were staying home.

But it wasn't completely empty. There was one other person there, who snapped a photo and sent it to *Expressen*.

Now Stefan Löfven had fallen into the trap, too.

Perhaps it was little by way of consolation, but during these weeks several of the prime minister's colleagues made similar mistakes. The minister for finance went on a ski trip, the minister for justice visited a shopping centre in Lund, and the director-general of the Swedish Civil Contingencies Agency went to the Canary Islands.

The representatives of the other parties weren't exactly more cunning.

In a phone interview on national radio, a member of parliament for the Moderates criticised the prime minister's shopping trip; a little later, it would emerge that she'd given the interview while on a visit to Spain. Belonging to the same party was the most powerful politician in Stockholm, Anna König Jerlmyr. Four days before Christmas, she chose to shut down all activities for children and young people, including outdoor ice rinks. 'I'm a parent with young children, too,' she said when the decision was made, 'so I can truly understand the frustration over a Christmas holiday without outdoor recreation.'

Then she got in her car and went on a ski trip with her family.

But all this was — as mentioned — nothing unusual. It was a type of political scandal arising in any country with tough restrictions.

Sweden had truly become a country like any other.

The only question was whether the error lay with the people or the restrictions.

A doctor returns

The final press conference of the year was held on 29 December. For some time now, the meetings had been held online. Now, decked out in gigantic headphones, Anders Tegnell tried in various ways to avoid commenting on the shopping habits of the prime minister or the minister for justice.

'Does walking into a shopping centre constitute an unnecessary risk?' someone asked.

'It depends on why you're going there,' the state epidemiologist answered.

'Is the recommendation still in place?' someone else wanted to know.

Yes, but the majority of the transmission was taking place at workplaces or in the home, so we mustn't forget what's most important.

Was he surprised that both the prime minister and the minister for justice had gone into shopping centres?

'We make no judgements about the actions of individuals.'

When the topic had been exhausted, the questions fell into a familiar pattern.

'Is it possible that infections are in fact even higher than the figures are showing?'

'Why aren't you analysing a larger portion of tests to identify new mutations?'

'The R number is above one! Why aren't you closing schools?'

'Why aren't you recommending face masks?'

Towards the end of the year, the questions had begun to change character. Ever since the second wave rolled in, Anders Tegnell had been forced to answer the same question — albeit phrased in different ways — more or less every day.

Why weren't they clamping down harder?

Why hadn't they introduced a lockdown? Why weren't schools

closing? Why were gyms still open? Why weren't they more worried about new variants? Why weren't Swedes forced to wear face masks? Why weren't entire families put into quarantine?

Anders Tegnell had different answers every time. Naturally. The questions were about different things.

His answers were detailed, and accounted for such things as effectiveness, timing, lack of resources for testing, immunity among the population, and the impact on children's health.

But, in truth, these were all versions of the same question: why weren't they doing more?

It was a peculiar situation. But it had been going on for so long that no one seemed to be reflecting on it.

The country's journalists — the ones who used to consider it their duty to protect their citizens' rights and liberties — asked Tegnell daily why he wasn't restricting their freedom of assembly, freedom of trade, or any other freedom considered until recently vital to democracy.

Several of the country's lawyers — the ones who'd go through the roof over someone being detained a few weeks too long — tweeted and wrote blog posts arguing that the constitution allowed for tougher restrictions than the government admitted. Lawyers who didn't agree on their interpretation wrote books saying that the constitution ought to be amended.

They begged to be imprisoned.

And Anders Tegnell resisted.

* * *

When the year was almost at an end, a Swedish doctor landed at a deserted Stockholm Arlanda Airport.

Johan von Schreeb had been away from home since August.

It was a long story. It had started when 2,750 tonnes of ammonium nitrate exploded in the port of Beirut. A hundred people died, 4,000 were injured, and the Swedish disaster doctor flew down to help.

But that was a whole other story. The kind that the year 2020 didn't quite have room for.

And now he was home again.

Returning to Sweden was always hard. It had been hard after Rwanda. And again after Sierra Leone.

This time was different. Not only because the situation had been under control by the time he made it down to Lebanon, and he'd thus been spared from seeing so much death and suffering this time.

This year, it was Sweden that was different. It felt naked, somehow. Unlike in Lebanon, Swedes generally walked around without face masks.

It felt nice that young people didn't seem to care about keeping their distance. It was sound.

Over the course of the days when he slowly acclimatised to Sweden again, he started thinking about something. The more Swedes he met, the more he began to wonder: did they realise how good they'd had it?

Did they realise what an asset it had been that schools had stayed open? That children had been allowed to go play at their friends' houses? That people had been allowed to meet up? That they had been allowed to play sports?

* * *

Around the same time, up in Umeå, another doctor sat there feeling nonplussed.

Just a few weeks earlier, Fredrik Elgh had believed Sweden was about to change tack. But after the heightened restrictions in November, almost nothing had happened.

In a few weeks, schools would reopen. Preschoolers, as well as students in year 1 to 6, would be allowed to see their classmates again.

Together with Björn Olsen, Åke Lundkvist, and several of the other scientists who for almost a year had been trying to change the minds of the Public Health Agency, the government — hell, Swedish public opinion in general — he was writing one more op-ed.

He had 29 co-authors this time. Their message was that schools shouldn't be allowed to reopen after the Christmas holiday. Couldn't they just stay closed for another four weeks? Two weeks?

But he had a feeling how it would end. On 11 January, schools would open again.

He really didn't understand.

But, he said, he was a pathologist and virologist. Not a psychologist. Not a political scientist.

'Perhaps the Swedish people like this. Perhaps this is what they want.'

* * *

Johan von Schreeb — the man who at the start of the year had trekked to the Public Health Agency, and in its dining hall had warned Anders Tegnell about the new virus — now feared other things entirely.

Why were the British letting the police fine them for going outside? Why weren't the French protesting? They, who'd protest just about anything?

It was fascinating. It was scary. The fears and processes being triggered were hard to resist.

There were larger questions than whether the Swedes in charge of infectious-disease control had been slow to act, whether their calculations were correct or not, whether their timelines for natural herd immunity and vaccine development had been accurate.

For what did the alternative to an open society look like?

He'd seen it, and he didn't like it.

Of course, Swedish society had been forced to pay a price, he thought. It was plain to see in the number of deaths, regardless of how you chose to read them.

Swedes had been allowed to live more freely than most. And more had died because of it.

And, just like that, 2020 was over.

Part VII

A year of freedom

On 6 March 2021, at 2.00 pm, a couple of hundred people gathered at the Medborgarplatsen square in Stockholm.

It was a heterogeneous group of people. They carried placards with messages critical of everything from the expansion of the 5G network to vaccination schemes and immigration policy. But they were all there to protest the restrictions placed on Swedish society.

One of those restrictions meant that freedom of assembly had temporarily been put on ice. Since the end of November, it had been prohibited to hold public gatherings with more than eight people.

Over the course of a few months, Swedish freedoms had gradually been curtailed — but without any real precision or consideration. It seemed more like the way a kebab shop might hack away at a gigantic hunk of meat on a stick in the course of a long day.

One little slice here; another slice there. A ban under the *Public Order Act* here; a restriction under the *Alcohol Act* there.

These changes had largely been pursued by the government, which had begun to override the Public Health Agency at an ever faster rate. But the restrictions were also being pushed by regional infectious-disease doctors, as well as local politicians and municipal department heads with the power to close indoor swimming pools and libraries, to recommend increased remote learning, and to introduce other measures.

The laws, regulations, and recommendations — both local and national — now governing the way Swedes lived their lives were so numerous that few could keep track of them all.

On 8 January, parliament had voted to approve the so-called pandemic law — a temporary act making it possible for the government to close gyms, indoor swimming pools, shops, and shopping centres. On 24 February, the same parliament had recommended that its members wear face masks in the chamber.

It was clear that the Swedish strategy was slowly being chipped away. Some even seemed to want to change the memory of it.

On the government's website, where since April 2020 it had said that 'the overall objective of the government's efforts is to reduce the pace of the Covid-19 virus's spread', the text was changed one day in late January 2021 to say that the goal was simply was to 'reduce the spread'.

The subordinate clause that used to follow — the one that read 'to "flatten the curve" so that large numbers of people do not become ill at the same time' — disappeared, too.

Once the change was discovered by the journalist Emanuel Karlsten, the government reverted to its original wording. The Government Offices maintained it had been a mistake.

Regardless of what happened, the Swedish shift was tangible.

Admittedly, there was still a gap between what was being imposed in Sweden and the rules that were in force in several other European countries. In France, 2 million people now lived under a form of 'weekend lockdown', and were prohibited from going outside on Saturdays and Sundays unless they had special reasons. Finland was headed into a three-week lockdown that involved closing restaurants. In England, there were certain criteria for when and how citizens were allowed to leave their homes. Germans in several states complained of having to wear face masks while jogging outside.

So far, no Swede had been prohibited from going outside — and once there, they were allowed to breathe however they liked. But from an international perspective, there were now several places that were a lot freer. A couple of days earlier, the state of Texas had practically opened up society completely again. Even the mask mandate was gone.

In Sweden, people were no longer allowed to demonstrate in the street in groups of more than eight.

So a few minutes after 2.00 pm on 6 March 2021, one of the police officers who had arrived at Medborgarplatsen gripped a microphone. His message poured forth from the speakers on a police car: 'Due to the high number of participants, in accordance with section 21 of the

Covid act, participants in this public gathering must immediately leave the scene.'

Instead, several protestors began to move north through the city toward the Kungsträdgården square, where they gathered once more.

A few minutes after 4.30 pm, it was all over. People dispersed; some were escorted away by the police. When the whole thing was over, six officers had been injured, one person had been arrested for blue-light sabotage, and a total of 50 people had been removed in accordance with the new law.

What happened in Stockholm that day was really nothing unusual. In Copenhagen, Berlin, London — in most European capitals — similar scenes had played out. What was unique about the Swedish demonstration was that it happened so late. There hadn't really been that much to protest.

The Swedish year of freedom had come to an end.

It had been one year to the day since Anders Tegnell sat in an empty dining hall at the Public Health Agency together with Denis Coulombier, Jan Albert, and Johan von Schreeb.

The path chosen at the time and over the following weeks turned Sweden into a control group for the enormous experiment the world was thrown into.

Sweden imposed no curfews, kept compulsory schools open, and didn't force its citizens to wear face masks.

The adjustments made to the strategy from November onward — both cosmetic and real — didn't succeed in wiping Sweden's unique path from memory. If anything, the opposite was true. When the Swedish parliament recommended face masks for its members no sooner than a year into the pandemic, it had the effect of highlighting the fact that for all this time members of parliament had *not* been masking up.

For almost all of 2020, Sweden had chosen a different path.

So, how did it go?

The results

It's no coincidence that the word 'viral' has gained new meaning in the digital age. Ideas, figures of thought, opinions — they spread the same way, from one person to another, and just as rapidly as the viruses the word originally referred to.

During the 2020 pandemic year, one such idea — one such thought — spread from country to country, from politician to politician. From China to Italy and Spain, across the European continent, to North America, South America, and Africa. It was the idea that countries could close down their societies, that by forcing people to stay home they could prevent the spread of the virus. It was an idea never before tested at such a scale, which had little support in science, and for which no one had calculated the social and economic costs.

But it was a powerful idea. And it spread.

In order to understand Sweden's actions in 2020, you have to forget for a moment about the medical, legal, and mathematical technicalities hashed over in detail on news shows, in the newspapers, and on social media.

Because, in truth, the people who — formally and informally — shaped the Swedish path through the initial months of the Covid-19 pandemic had different opinions about most things: about the spread of the virus at the start, about R numbers, about epidemiological models, about antibody studies, about the effectiveness of face masks, about the value of various recommendations. But there was one conviction they all shared: the virus wasn't as serious as the rest of the world believed.

Anders Tegnell, Johan Giesecke, Jan Albert, Tom Britton. They all made the assessment early on that the predictions that decision-makers in other countries were relying on — the ones warning of mass deaths and collapsing healthcare apparatuses — were wildly exaggerated.

In this, they had been right. There is no other conclusion to draw.

The report from Imperial College had predicted 510,000 deaths in the UK and 2.2 million in the US. When the year ended, around one-fifth as many had died — the exact figures depended, as always, on how the deaths were classified.

Tomas Pueyo's influential texts assumed a fatality rate of between 3.8 and 4.0 per cent. Judging by the increasingly thorough studies now being conducted in various countries, it was clear that the risk of dying if infected with the virus was significantly lower.

The calculation presented in April by scientists at Uppsala University, based on Imperial College's model, had warned that 96,000 Swedes would be dead by 1 July. When that date passed, fewer than a fifteenth of that number had died.

Anders Tegnell, Johan Giesecke, and Tom Britton had made a few erroneous predictions of their own: Tegnell, about the risk that the virus would make it to Sweden; Giesecke, about its deadliness being on a par with a regular seasonal flu; and Britton, about how quickly herd immunity would set in.

But the predictions shaping policies in the UK, France, the US, and several other countries had been significantly further from the actual outcome.

They had been more wrong.

When the number of deaths in the world ended up being lower than feared, some took it as proof that the restrictions had worked — that the extensive lockdowns had tamed the mortality. And that it could have been reduced even further if politicians had clamped down harder and sooner. To the British parliament, Neil Ferguson said that the UK could have halved its death toll if the lockdown had been initiated a week sooner.

But if so, the question of how to explain Sweden's figures remained. The country that, according to the outside world, had done everything wrong — the country that had been named a 'pariah state' by *The New York Times* — didn't just have a lower death toll per capita than the UK and the US. By the end of the year, most of Europe had worse figures. This was true whether measured in reported Covid deaths or excess mortality.

The US was perhaps the most interesting object of comparison.

Because of its political structure, the 50 states had chosen different paths through the pandemic: they had experienced different degrees of lockdown, been more or less ambitious about contact tracing, and been reached by the virus at different times.

California, the most populous state in the US, had initially appeared to be weathering the pandemic quite well. The virus reached it late, and the state governor, Gavin Newsom, imposed extensive restrictions on citizens' liberties. Schools closed. Beaches closed. An extensive testing apparatus was set in motion, too. Already in early May, 35,000 tests were carried out per day.

Throughout the spring, both the rate of transmission and the number of deaths had remained low. But eventually the virus hit. And by early 2021 California had almost exactly as many Covid deaths — per capita — as Sweden. The same pattern could be seen across the country.

If Sweden had been a US state, ranked by deaths per capita, it would have come in somewhere around 30th place. And half of America's children still had no school to go to.

When the history books were closed on the year 2020, the total figure was 98,124. That's how many people died in Sweden in 2020.

It was a lot more than in previous years. The annual average for the years 2015 to 2019 had been 90,962 people.

But it was almost exactly as many as had died in 1993. That year, 97,008 deaths had been recorded by Statistics Sweden.

Taking into account that Sweden's population was a lot smaller in the early 1990s than now, 1993 appeared worse. Comparatively, a smaller portion of the population had died in 2020.

On the other hand, medical advancements and improved living conditions achieved over the 27 years between 1993 and 2020 had pushed down mortality figures so much that it was perhaps reasonable to expect a structurally lower mortality.

There was a lot to discuss. But the overall conclusion was irrefutable: the pandemic that had struck Sweden was no historical anomaly. It was no storm of the century, no new Spanish flu.

The year 2020 had been a bit like the year 1993. A deadly month in 2020 had been like a deadly month in 1993.

And above all: Sweden had got off easier than several of the countries that had closed down early and hard.

* * *

Comparing death tolls, examining the effectiveness of lockdowns, was a politically sensitive issue to say the least. All over the world, powerful politicians — many with brilliant careers ahead of them — had curtailed the liberties of their citizens. They had denied children months of in-person schooling — in several cases, a whole year's worth of teaching.

But for what gain?

The same politicians had spent enormous sums on testing and contact-tracing their populations. The use of these programs, too, was highly unclear.

It was no secret that Anders Tegnell and Johan Giesecke felt the world had rushed headlong into rugged terrain in the spring of 2020.

It was 'mad', as Tegnell wrote to his confidants.

It was a world governed with 'little wisdom', according to Giesecke.

When the final results were in, no other conclusion could be drawn.

By the time the pandemic was more than a year old, several studies were published that showed lockdowns had had a limited impact — if any — on the numbers of people who had died of Covid.

At the same time, the costs of lockdowns were beginning to show. When the US Census Bureau asked Americans how they were feeling at the end of 2020, 42 per cent responded that they were suffering from anxiety or depression. This marked an increase from 11 per cent the year before. In Denmark, scientists had followed 11 schoolchildren from the same class throughout the pandemic. During the year, the children — who were in eighth grade — gained an average of 7.6 kilos (18.8 pounds), of which 3.3 kilos (7.3 pounds) was pure fat. According to the UNICEF, the situation for the world's children had regressed on all measurable indicators.

According to the World Bank, the number of people living in extreme poverty was expected to rise for the first time in 20 years. This fate was now estimated to afflict between 88 million and 115 million people.

Sweden had not been spared. For much of 2020, the country's students in upper-secondary school had been denied in-person teaching. At the beginning of 2021, students in yeasr 6 to 9 in several municipalities had been affected, too.

But in most respects, Sweden had been saved from the devastation afflicting societies that had shut down. The primary schools for years 1 to 3 and for years 4 to 6 had stayed open. Parks and beaches had remained open. Everyone had retained their legal right to move freely within the country. With a few exceptions, youth sports had been allowed to continue. No Swede had ever been prohibited from leaving their house. No Swede had ever been forced to wear a face mask outside.

Despite the Swedish government now trying to make it appear as though Sweden hadn't in fact chosen a different path, the truth was that Sweden had been a freer country. And it had worked.

'Choose you must, and die you must'

The dilemma plaguing the world in 2020 was really the same that it had wrestled with 300 years earlier: what risk should you expose the population to?

The thinkers of the eighteenth century had to choose between exposing people to the risks of immunisation and the risks of being receptive to the smallpox virus.

The politicians of the twenty-first century had to choose between allowing some transmission of the new, largely unknown virus, to allow the functions of society to continue, and shutting down society to lower the risk of infection.

Those choosing the latter — the lockdown path — often referred to the precautionary principle: faced with an unknown situation, it was a safer option.

But which was the more cautious path? Shutting down all of society in a way that had never before been tested? Or waiting? A choice had to be made. There was no escaping it.

Through cold, mathematical analysis, the smallpox choice was made a little simpler in the 1700s: it was clear that human lives could be saved if you accepted that some people would die from immunisation.

When Sweden made its choice in 2020, it happened the same way.

By calculation.

Three central assumptions lay behind that calculation: that the fatality rate was a lot lower than the figures circulating at the start of the pandemic, that lockdowns did more harm than good, and that a growing immunity — regardless of whether or not you chose to call it herd immunity — would sooner or later be what protected the population.

Tegnell & co. ended up being right about the first two. But the final assumption was more complicated to evaluate. By the time the second wave hit Europe, much of what Johan Giesecke had predicted on his digital spring tour of the continent had indeed come true: many of the countries that hadn't been affected in the spring — Germany, the Czech Republic, Hungary, Estonia — and thus lacked immunity, recorded high numbers of infection during the autumn.

But then came the vaccines. And by the time spring arrived in 2021, it was clear that it would largely be vaccinations — not a naturally acquired herd immunity — that would pave the way out of the pandemic. Yet in several countries — including the US and the UK — the number of cases and deaths had started to drop before mass vaccinations were initiated.

They'd been right two and a half times out of three.

The basic analysis of the situation that Anders Tegnell and Johan Giesecke acted on from the middle of March 2020 — and which was largely shared by Jan Albert, Tom Britton, Johan von Schreeb, Matti Sällberg, and others — was in no way unique. At universities and government agencies all over the world, other epidemiologists, doctors, mathematicians, and statisticians were interpreting the early data in similar ways.

But after the publication of the Imperial College report, after the 'hammer and the dance', after the wave of lockdowns starting in mid-March, it became increasingly difficult to question the policies applied.

The fact that critics in several cases were censored by large American platform companies was perhaps less significant than the way in which, early on, influential journalistic institutions in the US and Europe — such as *The New York Times*, the *BBC*, *The Guardian*, *The New Yorker*, and *The Atlantic*, as well as the big German media outlets — chose to equate those who expressed lockdown scepticism with a general contempt for science. When German, Danish, or Norwegian media outlets reported on Sweden's chosen path, it was like they were describing a banana republic.

Throughout 2020, it remained difficult to argue for any other solution than the one so many countries had chosen. Scientists who did so suffered badly: they saw their invitations to conferences withdrawn; their institutions distanced themselves from them.

In this respect, too, Sweden was an exception. The debate about what level of restrictions should apply was perhaps louder than in other countries — but it was also freer.

It wasn't so strange that this debate turned harsh. As the virus swept through Sweden, new winners and losers were created in society.

A seven-year-old was allowed to go to school, eat school lunches, and see their friends every day.

A seventy-year-old, however, was advised to stay home.

During the year-long debate about Sweden's actions, several voices accused the Swedish constitution of being outdated. They said the government lacked the powers to respond to a pandemic, that the Swedish administrative model, with its independent government agencies, wasn't working in today's society.

The problem with this analysis was that it assumed there were key interventions that those in power wanted to impose — but couldn't.

But the strategy pursued by Anders Tegnell — and which the government accepted in full until mid-November — was in all respects the one he wanted to pursue.

Compulsory schools stayed open because they were supposed to be open, not because of some defect in the constitution. The Swedes were free because they were supposed to be free.

That was the calculation they'd made.

'Choose you must. And die you must.'

Once again, Johan Giesecke sat in front of his computer in the same study where, in January 2020, he'd read about a new virus from China.

That was only 15 months ago, but it felt longer. The second Covid winter had been colder than the first. The lake outside his window had frozen over and melted again. The swim season was over for both him and his wife.

'These are the only musts in life.'

It was one of those things he liked to say. Choose and die. Really, the moral was something like, *You shouldn't get all up in arms over worldly things*. But, over the past year, the old epidemiologist's maxim had gained new meaning.

Everyone had been given a choice.

There never had been a cautious, risk-free alternative. There never was a path that guaranteed less death, less suffering, than any other. There only ever were different alternatives carrying different risks.

The choice that Sweden had made was clear. But it was also unspoken.

Now, long into the pandemic, Johan Giesecke dared to speak about that choice. With every passing day, with every interview he did, his sentences grew plainer and plainer. Clearer and clearer.

It was really quite simple: his life, he argued, was less valuable than his grandchildren's lives. And not just his grandchildren's. All children's lives.

Their opportunities to get an education, to grow, were more important than reducing the risk of him — now 71 years old — being infected with the virus.

The deaths among the country's elderly — yes, this was a sorrow they'd have to carry with them for a long time. But these were the terms.

Every nation had been forced to choose a path.

And Sweden had chosen its.

Epilogue

A hundred years ago, a big demonstration took place in New York City. It was a summer's day in 1921. It was 4 July, to be exact — the United States' Independence Day.

Between 2.00 and 4.00 pm, 20,000 people marched down Fifth Avenue. They sang, chanted, and waved placards in the air. One of them featured Leonardo da Vinci's painting *The Last Supper*, bearing the words: 'Wine was served'.

'Tyranny in the name of righteousness is the basest of all tyranny,' read another.

'Hooray for the beer,' yelled a grey-haired woman, according to a *New York Times* article the next day.

What transpired that day was the result of one of the biggest experiments in public health policy ever conducted. For a year, beer, wine, and spirits had been illegal throughout the United States. In an amendment to the US constitution, all production, transport, and sales of alcohol had been banned.

From a public health perspective, it seemed a reasonable step to take. That alcohol was a dangerous substance was clear enough: disease, violence, poverty, and crime were intimately bound up with the drug.

As so often in the history of democracy, the Americans now found themselves wrestling with the balance between freedom and security. Was it really right to prevent a free people from making beverages they not only enjoyed, but which also served important cultural and religious purposes?

The protestors marching south through Manhattan that day had no doubt in their minds: this was an anti-democratic artifice. Their placards referred to George Washington, Thomas Jefferson, and Abraham Lincoln. This was no way to govern a free country.

Twelve years later, the experiment ended. In 1933, alcohol became legal again.

But it wasn't because the libertarian arguments had won out. It wasn't because those protestors suddenly gained sympathy for their opinions.

Nor was it because the drug itself was considered less harmful to people's health.

The reason Prohibition came to an end was that it simply didn't work.

It no longer mattered all that much whether alcohol was harmful or not. It made no difference what political opinions people held.

If it didn't work, then it didn't work.

Because, regardless of what the law said, Americans didn't stop consuming alcohol. The drinking simply moved from bars to 'speakeasies'. People learned to brew their own spirits. Smuggling in alcohol from Canada turned into a national pastime. And the American mafia gained a new source of revenue.

Today, most agree that this experiment — the 'noble experiment', as American historians like to call it — was a gigantic failure.

Until just over two years ago, Prohibition remained the biggest experiment in social engineering ever undertaken by a democracy.

But then the year 2020 came along.

A new virus began to seep out of China. And the world initiated a new experiment.

Faced with this threat, the governments of the world came up with a whole new set of measures to stop the spread. By closing schools, banning people from gathering, forcing entrepreneurs to shut their businesses, and making their citizens wear face masks, the idea was that lives could be saved.

Just like the 'noble experiment' in the US, this too sparked debate. In all the democracies around the world, freedom was weighed against what was seen as security; individual rights stood against what was considered best for public health.

The path that Sweden chose through the pandemic stood out in several ways. To its citizens, this was most clear in that they generally didn't have to wear face masks, young children continued going to school, and leisure activities were largely allowed to go on unhindered.

Some groups saw their lives or livelihoods disproportionally curtailed:

upper-secondary-school students, people over the age of 70, restaurant workers.

But there was no question about it — Swedes lived more freely than others.

Eleven years after that demonstration in New York, the US Supreme Court ruled in a case known as *New State Ice Co. v. Liebmann*.

It had nothing to do with alcohol. It didn't concern anything all that interesting today. It was about whether Oklahoma had a right to require that companies selling ice within the state hold a special licence.

No, the court declared. Anyone who wanted to could sell ice.

That was that. And in all likelihood, this obscure dispute would quickly have fallen into oblivion if it weren't for the dissenting opinion written and filed by one of the nine judges.

The judge's name was Louis Brandeis, and he wanted to draw the other jurists' attention to what he called a 'happy incident' in American democracy.

'A single courageous State,' he wrote, 'may, if its citizens choose, serve as a laboratory; and try novel social and economic experiments without risk to the rest of the country.'

The year was 1932, and Brandeis recounted the revolutionary scientific leaps recently produced by the West: 'The discoveries in physical science, the triumphs in invention, attest the value of the process of trial and error. In large measure, these advances have been due to experimentation.'

So why should a democracy divest itself of the same opportunity to learn, to advance, to improve the lives of its citizens?

To experiment, simply put.

Since then, Brandeis's figure of thought has come to be known as the 'laboratories of democracy'. If you are a political scientist you may prefer to call it 'institutional competition', but its essence remains the same: bad ideas are eliminated and gradually replaced by better ones. Thanks to the failed American experiment with a ban on alcohol, no other democracy has tried it since.

They conducted an experiment. And we learned from it.

* * *

During the first six months of the pandemic, the word 'experiment' had a negative ring to it. For that's what the Swedes were subjecting themselves to when they — compared to the rest of the world — maintained some semblance of normality.

This experiment was quickly condemned by the outside world as a failure.

You could say that a hypothesis was formulated; it maintained that the freedom in Sweden would be costly.

The absence of restrictions, open schools, reliance on recommendations instead of mandates and police enforcement would all result in a higher death toll than in other countries. Meanwhile, the lack of freedom endured by citizens elsewhere would save lives.

At this stage, it was not unreasonable to assume that Sweden would pay a high price for its freedom. In the US, with its forceful lockdowns, the death toll per capita was significantly lower than in Sweden throughout the spring of 2020. And on sites where the ravages of the pandemic could be followed in real time — such as Our World in Data, the Johns Hopkins University database, or Worldometer — it was clear that Sweden had more deaths per capita than most other countries.

But the experiment went on. During the months that followed, the virus continued to ravage the world, and the death toll in several of the countries that had locked down began to surpass Sweden's — one by one.

The UK, the US, France, Poland, Portugal, Hungary, Spain, Argentina, Belgium — countries that had shut down playgrounds, forced children to wear face masks, closed schools, fined citizens for hanging out on the beach, and surveilled parks with drones — were all hit harder than Sweden.

When the European statistics agency Eurostat measured excess mortality for the whole of 2020, Sweden ended up in 22nd place out of 30 European countries. In a report by the UK Office for National Statistics, which adjusted the results for such factors as age structure, Sweden ranked 18th out of 26.

And the pandemic was far from over.

***

In December 2021, the second year of the pandemic was coming to an end. And in Sweden, most things had gone back to normal again.

The Allsvenskan football league finals were played in front of a full stadium. People went to work. Buses and trains were busy once more.

On the quiet, the Swedish pandemic had entered a new phase.

After roughly six months of various — albeit relatively light — restrictions, Sweden was for the most part free again.

University students had returned to large lecture halls, night clubs were open, cinemas became more and more crowded. The biggest difference compared to a regular year was that entrance into events with more than 100 participants required proof of vaccination.

Once again, this new phase was characterised by Swedes enjoying freedoms that citizens of other countries were denied. And still, almost no one wore a face mask.

Once again, Sweden stuck out. But there were no longer any foreign journalists at the Public Health Agency's press conferences. No Americans, Brits, Germans, or Danes asked why schools were staying open, or why the country hadn't gone into lockdown.

In large part, it was because the rest of the world had quietly begun to live with the new virus. Most of the world's politicians had given up hope on both lockdowns and school closures.

But they could have asked about the absence of face masks. British and Danish journalists could have questioned why the Swedes still carried out so little testing compared to the agencies in their own countries.

It was a little strange, really. Considering all those articles and TV segments that had been produced the year before about Sweden's foolishly libertarian attitude to the pandemic, considering the way some data sources had been referenced daily by the world's media, it appeared as though the same sources were now of no interest whatsoever.

For anyone still interested, the results were impossible to deny. By the end of 2021, 56 countries had registered more deaths per capita from Covid-19 than Sweden.

And when the UK Office for National Statistics updated their figures, it turned out that during the period of just under 18 months between January 2020 and June 2021, Sweden had experienced an excess mortality of minus 2.3 per cent. Together with seven other European countries — including its three Nordic neighbours — Sweden had actually experienced a mortality deficit during the pandemic.

With regard to the restrictions that the rest of the world had put so much faith in — school closures, lockdowns, face masks, mass testing — Sweden had more or less gone in the opposite direction.

Yet these were the results.

There were, of course, other possible ways to measure the ravages of the pandemic: the prevalence of post-viral syndrome in society (commonly referred to as 'long Covid'); an increased budget deficit; unemployment; and so on.

Yet Sweden couldn't be said to stand out on the basis of these measures either.

It was beginning to become increasingly clear that the political measures that had been deployed against the virus were of limited value.

But about this, no one spoke.

From a human perspective, it was easy to understand the reluctance to face the numbers from Sweden. For the inevitable conclusion must be that millions of people had lived unfreely, and millions of children had had their education disrupted — all for naught.

Who would want to be complicit in that?

Yet the laboratories of democracy had carried out their human experiments. And the results were clear.

Exactly why it turned out this way is harder to explain. But perhaps the 'noble experiment' of the 1920s in the US can offer some clues.

Back then, the mistake the American authorities made was to underestimate the complexity of society. Just because they banned alcohol, it didn't mean alcohol disappeared. People's drives, desires, and behaviours were impossible to predict, impossible to suppress by planning.

A hundred years later, many of those in power made the same mistake. Simply closing schools didn't stop children from meeting in other settings. When the same decision-makers shut down life in the cities, those who could do so relocated to their vacation homes, spreading the infection to new places. The authorities urged their citizens to buy food online, without thinking more closely about who would transport the goods from place to place.

If the politicians had been honest with themselves, they might have foreseen what would happen. Because, just like during Prohibition — when American politicians were constantly caught drinking alcohol — a hundred years later, their successors were caught breaking precisely the restrictions they had imposed on everyone else.

The mayors of New York and Chicago, the US Speaker of the House, the British government's top advisor, the Dutch minister of justice, the EU's trade commissioner, the governor of California, the prime minister of Finland — the list grew ever longer.

It's hard to plan other people's lives. It's hard to dictate desirable behaviours in a population. This is a lesson many dictators have learned. During the Covid-19 pandemic, many democracies have learned it, too. Perhaps the lesson has not yet sunk in, but it might eventually.

Then perhaps it will be another hundred years before we make the same mistake again.

Acknowledgements

Several people have assisted me with translations, chasing down books, research, medical reasoning, mathematical questions, and other issues arising during the course of the work. Thanks to John Karlsson Valik, Philip Gerlee, Lina Lund, Ossi Kurki-Suonio, Torbjörn Nilsson, Karin Ström, Max-Jedeur Palmgren, Lia Fallenius, Svante Weyler, Ingmar Neveus, Anders Billing, Mattias Axelsson, and Ania Obminska.

Jesper Högström read innumerable drafts, and was a source of support in my work more or less daily for a whole year. Thank you.

Bibliography

The material in this book is largely based on publicly available sources: email conversations, internal documents, meeting minutes, newspaper articles, et cetera. The great majority of that material is public — in the sense that anyone could request it — but I have also had access to several documents not covered by the Swedish principle of public access to official records.

The representations herein are also based on a couple of hundred interviews with people who have in some way had insight into the sequence of events or the characters in the drama.

The sources listed in the bibliography are the ones I have either cited or relied on for any information I haven't produced myself.

The book was fact-checked by Johannes Eimer.

Books/Articles

Abbott, Allison. 'Covid's Mental-Health Toll: how scientists are tracking a surge in depression'. *Nature*. 2021-02-03.

Andersson, Fredrik N.G., and Jonung, Lars. 'Nedstängningar står inte på vetenskaplig grund' (Lockdowns lack support in science). *Dagens Industri*. 2021-03-11.

Andersson, Ulrika. 'Stort förtroende för Folkhälsomyndigheten och 1177 under coronapandemin' (High confidence in the Public Health Agency and 1177 during the Covid-19 pandemic). Gothenburg, Sweden: The SOM Institute & Gothenburg University, 2020.

Andersson, Warwick. 'Immunities of Empire: race, disease, and the new tropical medicine, 1900–1920'. *Bulletin of the History of Medicine*. Vol. 70, no. 1, 1996: 94–118.

Associated Press. 'China Didn't Warn Public of Likely Pandemic for 6 Key Days'. 2020-04-15.

Atterstam, Inger. 'Massvaccinering räddade sex liv' (Mass vaccination saved six lives). *Svenska Dagbladet*. 2012-02-15.

Baldwin, Peter. *Contagion and the State in Europe, 1830–1930*. Cambridge University Press, 1999.

———. *Fighting the First Wave*. Cambridge University Press, 2021.

Bendavid, Eran; Oh, Christopher; Bhattacharya, Jay and Ioannidis, John. 'Assessing Mandatory Stay-at-Home and Business Closure Effects on the Spread of Covid-19'. *Public Health*. 2021.

Benedelle, Cecilia, and Westling, Fanny. 'Europeiska kvinnor flyr karantänen — för att lyxfesta i Stockholm' (European women flee quarantine — to attend luxury parties in Stockholm). *Aftonbladet*. 2020-04-18.

Bergstedt, Therese. 'Folkhälsomyndigheten: Utred förbudet att ta droger' (The Public Health Agency: investigate the ban on using drugs). *SVT Nyheter*. 2020-05-08.

Bernoulli, Daniel and Blower, Sally. 'An Attempt at a New Analysis of the Mortality Caused by Smallpox and of the Advantages of Inoculation to Prevent It.' *Reviews in Medical Virology*. Vol. 14, no. 5, 2004: 275–288.

Bethge, Philip; Elger, Katrin; Glüsing, Jens; Grill, Markus; Hackenbrock, Veronika; Puhl, Jan; von Rohr, Mathieu; and Traufetter, Gerald. 'Reconstruction of a Mass Hysteria: the swine flu panic of 2009'. Trans. Christopher Sultan. *Spiegel International*. 2010-03-12.

Bhattacharya, Jay and Kulldorff, Martin. 'The Case Against Covid Tests for the Young and Healthy'. *The Wall Street Journal*. 2020-09-03.

Bosman, Julie and Tompkins, Lucy. 'Texas Drops Its Virus Restrictions as a Wave of Reopenings Takes Hold'. *The New York Times*. 2021-03-02.

Bostock, Bill. 'How "Professor Lockdown" Helped Save Tens of Thousands of Lives Worldwide — and Carried Covid-19 into Downing Street'. *Business Insider*. 2020-04-25.

Bower, Tom. *Boris Johnson: The Gambler*. Random House, 2020

Branswell, Helen. 'A Severe Flu Season Is Stretching Hospitals Thin. That Is a Very Bad Omen'. *STAT News*. 2018-01-15.

Bratt, Anna. 'Lyckad vaccination sparar 2,5 miljarder' (Successful vaccination saves 2.5 billion SEK). *Dagens Nyheter*. 2009-09-18.

Brauer, Fred. 'Mathematical Epidemiology: past, present, and future'. *Infectious Disease Modelling*. Vol. 2, no. 2, 2017: 113–127.

Britton, Tom; Ball, Frank; and Trapman, Pieter. 'A Mathematical Model Reveals the Influence of Population Heterogeneity on Herd Immunity to SARS-CoV-2'. *Science*. 2020-06-23.

Brouwers, Lisa; Cakici, Baki; Camitz, Martin; Tegnell, Anders; and Boman, Magnus. 'Economic Consequences to Society of Pandemic H1N1 Influenza 2009 — preliminary results for Sweden'. *Eurosurveillance*. 2009.

Calvert, Jonathan; Arbuthnott, George; Das, Shanti; Calver, Tom; and Russell-Jones, Lily. '48 Hours in September When Ministers and Scientists Split over Covid Lockdown'. *The Times*. 2020-12-13.

Chang, I-wei Jennifer. 'Taiwan's Model for Combating Covid-19: a small island with big data'. *Mei at 75*. 2020-11-10.

Chaudhry, Rabail; Dranitsaris, George; Mulbashir, Talha; Bartoszko, Justyna; and Riazi, Sheila. 'A Country Level Analysis Measuring the Impact of Government Actions, Country Preparedness and Socioeconomic Factors on Covid-19 Mortality and Related Health Outcomes'. *The Lancet*. 2020-07-21.

Christakis, Nicholas A. *Apollo's Arrow*. Little, Brown and Company, 2020.

Cowley, Jason. 'Neil Ferguson: the Covid modeler'. *New Statesman*. 2020-07-31.

Dahlager, Lars. 'Tog vi fejl om flokimmunitet? De meget lave svenske smittetal tyder på det' (Were we wrong about herd immunity? Very low Swedish infection rates suggest so). *Politiken*. 2020-09-17.

Delin, Mikael. 'Statsepidemiolog Anders Tegnell: Sverige har väldigt svårt att acceptera risker' (State epidemiologist Anders Tegnell: Sweden has a very hard time accepting risk). *Dagens Nyheter*. 2020-03-11.

Dietz, Klaus and Heesterbeek, J.A.P. 'Daniel Bernoulli's Epidemiological Model Revisited'. *Mathematical Biosciences*. Vol. 180, no. 1–2, 2002: 1–21.

Dimichele, Angie. 'Desantis Roundtable on Public Health'. *The Herald Tribune*. 2020-09-24.

Eidebo Berg, Jennifer. 'Europeisk rekommendation om munskydd vid tågresor' (European recommendation about face masks on trains). *TT News Agency*. 2020-07-21.

Elgh, Fredrik. 'Vi bör förbereda oss för ett värsta scenario' (We should prepare for a worst-case scenario). *Svenska Dagbladet*. 2020-03-02.

Eriksson, Göran; Pirttisalo Sallininen; Jani and Reuterskiöld, Annie. 'Så föddes Sveriges coronaplan — spelet bakom kulisserna' (How Sweden's Covid plan was born — the drama behind the scenes). *Svenska Dagbladet*. 2020-07-05.

Ewald, Hugo. 'Anders Tegnell: Ingen andra våg i Sverige' (Anders Tegnell: no second wave in Sweden). *Dagens Nyheter*. 2020-10-15.

Eyler, John M. 'The Changing Assessments of John Snow's and William Farr's Cholera Studies'. *Soz Praventivmed*. Vol. 46, no. 4 (2001): 225–32.

Ferguson, Neil M.; Keeling, Matt J.; Edmunds, W. John; Gani, Raymond; Grenfell, Bryan T.; Anderson, Roy M.; and Leach, Steve. 'Planning for Smallpox Outbreaks'. *Nature*. 2003-10-16.

Ferguson, Neil M.; Laydon, Daniel; Nedjati-Gilani, Gemma; et al. 'Report 9: Impact of non-pharmaceutical interventions (NPIs) to reduce Covid-19 mortality and healthcare demand'. Imperial College London. 2020-03-16.

Fine, Paul; Eames, Ken; and Heyman, David L. '"Herd Immunity": A Rough Guide'. *Clinical Infectious Diseases*. Vol. 52, no. 7 (2011): 911–916.

Fink, Sheri. 'White House Takes New Line after Dire Report on Death Toll. *New York Times*. 2020-03-16.

Frans, Emma. *Alla tvättar händerna* (Everybody wash their hands). Volante, 2021.

Friberg, Jacob. 'Mail afslører: Søren Brostrøm frarådede at lukke skoler kort før pressemøde' (Mail reveals: Søren Brostrøm advised against closing schools shortly before press conference). *BT*. 2020-07-24.

Funkquist, Matilda. 'Vård som tvång' (Forced care). Dissertation. Faculty of Law, Lund University, 2013.

Gardner, Jasmine; Willem, Lander; Van der Wijngaart, Kamerlin; Wouter, Shina Caroline Lynn; Brusselaers, Nele; and Kasson, Peter. 'Intervention Strategies Against Covid-19 and Their Estimated Impact on Swedish Healthcare Capacity'. *medRxiv*. 2020-04-11.

Gaudilliére, Jean-Paul and Löwy, Ilana. *Heredity and Infection: the history of disease transmission*. Routledge, 2015.

Giesecke, Johan. 'Lyssna inte på läkarvetenskapen' (Don't listen to the medical sciences). *Dagens Nyheter*. 1992-04-03.

———. *Modern Infectious Disease Epidemiology*. Routledge, 2017.

Gleeson, Colin. 'Swedish Expert Backtracks on Herd Immunity for Ireland'. *The Irish Times*. 2020-09-23.

Gorvett, Zaria. 'The Tricky Politics of Naming the New Coronavirus'. *BBC Future*, 2020-02-17.

Hamlin, C. 'Could You Starve to Death in England in 1839? The Chadwick–

Farr controversy and the loss of the "social" in public health'. *American Journal of Public Health.* Vol. 85, no. 6, 1995: 856–66.

Hanson, Matilda E. and Atterstam Inger. 'Läkarna måste inse att detta är politik och affärer' (Doctors must realise this is politics and business). *Svenska Dagbladet.* 2020-02-12.

Hedin, Björn. 'Debattörer riskerar förtroendet för forskarvärlden' (Debaters putting confidence in research world at risk). *Ny Teknik.* 2020-04-20.

Hedlund, Ingvar. 'Dödshemmet' (The death home). *Expressen.* 1994-03-15.

Hedrich, A.W. 'Monthly Estimates of the Child Population "Susceptible" to Measles, 1900–1931'. *American Journal of Epidemiology.* Vol. 17, no. 3, 1933: 613–636.

Heneghan, Carl and Jefferson, Tom. 'Covid-19: William Farr's way out of the pandemic'. The Centre for Evidence-Based Medicine, University of Oxford. 2020-04-11.

Hennel, Lena and Olsson, Lova. *Humlan som flyger. Berättelsen om Stefan Löfven* (The bumblebee flies: the story of Stefan Löfven). Norstedts, 2013.

Heyman, Eva. 'Döda på golvet i överfulla bårhus' (Dead lie on the floor in overflowing morgues). *Göteborgs-Posten.* 1994-01-14.

Hirschfeldt, Johan and Petersson, Olof. *Rättsregler i kris* (Legal rules in crisis). Dialogos, 2020.

Hjertén, Linda. 'Fältsjukhuset i Älvsjö avvecklas — användes aldrig' (Älvsjö field hospital discontinued — never used). *Dagens Nyheter.* 2020-06-04.

Holm, Gusten. 'Tegnells fel i bråket med de 22 forskarna' (Tegnell's error in the fight with the 22 scientists). *Expressen.* 2020-04-24.

Holm, Gusten; Sohl Stjernberg, Max; Ingmo, Daniel; and Lundberg Andersson, Hannes. 'Bilderna avslöjar: här julbesöker Löfven Gallerian' (Images reveal: Löfven on Christmas visit to shopping centre). *Expressen.* 2020-12-29.

Holmström, Mikael. 'Över en halv miljon danskar bedöms kunna smittas av nya coronaviruset' (Estimates indicate more than half a million Danes may become infected with novel coronavirus). *Dagens Nyheter.* 2020-03-11.

Ioannidis, John P.A. 'A Fiasco in the Making? As the coronavirus pandemic takes hold, we are making decisions without reliable data'. *Statnews.* 2020-03-17.

———. 'Infection Fatality Rate of Covid-19 Inferred from Seroprevalence Data'. *Bulletin of the World Health Organization.* 2020-10-14.

————. 'Why Most Published Research Findings Are False'. *PloS Medicine*. Vol. 2, no. 8, 2005: e124.

Jakobson, Hanna. 'Folkhälsomyndigheten: 10.000-15.000 kan bli sjuka i värsta fall' (Public Health Agency: at worst 10,000–15,000 may fall ill). *Dagens Nyheter*. 2020-03-03.

————. 'Löfven: Coronakommission tillsätts innan sommaren' (Löfven: Covid-19 commission appointed before summer). *Dagens Nyheter*. 2020-06-01.

Janssen, Marijn; Wimmer, Maria A.; and Deljoo, A., eds. *Policy Practice and Digital Science*. Springer International Publishing. 2015.

Jansson, Anders. 'Livsfarliga råd till vården och samhället om risker med coronaviruset' (Life-threatening advice to the healthcare services and society about risks of coronavirus). *Läkartidningen*. 2020-03-05.

Kalling, Lars O. *Det passionerade sändebudet* (The passionate messenger). *Carlssons förlag*, 2016.

Kelly, Jemima. 'That Imperial Coronavirus Report, in Detail'. *Financial Times*. 2020-03-16.

Karlsten, Emanuel. 'Mejlen som avslöjar Gieseckes inflytande' (Emails reveal Giesecke's influence). *Expressen*. 2020-08-11.

Klein, Daniel B.; Book, Joakim; and Bjørnskov, Christian. '16 Possible Factors for Sweden's High Covid Death Rate Among the Nordics'. GMU Working Paper in Economics No. 20–27, 14 August 2020.

Knowles, Megan. 'San Diego Hospital Opens Surge Tent After Area Flu Cases Quadruple'. *Becker's Hospital Review*. 2017-12-28.

Koffmar, Linda. 'Forskare tar fram modell för virusspridning i Sverige' (Researchers model spread of virus in Sweden). Uppsala University. 2020-04-02.

Kolata, Gina. *Flu: the story of the great influenza pandemic of 1918 and the search for the virus that caused it*. Touchstone, 2001.

Kristersson, Ulf and Svantesson, Elisabeth. 'Sverige behöver exitstrategi för återstart av ekonomin' (Sweden needs exit strategy for restarting the economy). *Dagens Nyheter*. 2020-04-28.

Kronqvist, Patrik. 'Världen bör räkna med fler pandemier från Kina' (The world should expect more pandemics from China). *Expressen*. 2020-03-26.

Kulldorff, Martin; Huang, Lan; Pickle, Linda; and Duczmal, Luis. 'An Elliptic Spatial Scan Statistic'. *Stat Med*. Vol. 25, no. 22, 2006: 3929–43.

Landler, Mark and Castle, Stephen. 'Britain Placed Under a Virtual Lockdown by Boris Johnson'. *The New York Times*. 23-03-2020.

Larsson, Petter J. 'Anders Tegnell hyllar brittisk tanke kring flockimmunitet: "Dit vi behöver komma"' (Anders Tegnell praises British idea of herd immunity: 'where we need to get'). *Aftonbladet*. 2020-03-16.

Liljebäck, Palle. 'Tom räknar på smittspridning' (Tom calculates spread of infection). *Naturvetarna*. 2020-03-30.

Lindstedt, Gunnar. 'Fem frågor om smittspridningen i Wuhan som Kina vägrat besvara' (Five questions about the spread of virus in Wuhan that China has refused to answer). *Fokus*. 2020-05-20.

Lindström, Olle. 'Finansministern: Man förhandlar inte med virus' (Finance minister: there is no negotiating with a virus). *TT News Agency*. 2020-03-20.

Liu, Jie; Xie, Wanli; Wang, Yanting; Xiong, Yue; Chen, Shiqiang; Han, Jingjing; and Wua, Qingping. 'A Comparative Overview of Covid-19, MERS and SARS: review article'. *International Journal of Surgery*. Vol. 81, 2020: 1–8.

Ludvigsson, Jonas F. 'Ett skolboksexempel på modellers tillkortakommande' (A textbook example of shortcomings of modelling). *Dagens Nyheter*. 2020-04-15.

———. 'Medicinskt detektivarbete löste koleragåtan' (Medical detective work solved the cholera mystery). *Svenska Dagbladet*. 2020-08-26.

Lundberg, Anna. *Läkarnas blanka vapen: svensk smittskyddslagstiftning i historiskt perspektiv* (The physicians' shining sword: Swedish infectious disease legislation in a historical perspective). Nordic Academic Press, 2016.

Lundh, Torbjörn and Gerlee, Philip. *Vetenskapliga modeller: svarta lådor, röda atomer och vita lögner* (Scientific models: black boxes, red atoms and white lies). Studentlitteratur, 2012.

Luque Fernandez, Miguel A.; Schomaker, Michael; Mason, Peter R.; Fesselet, Jean F.; Baudot, Yves; Boulle, Andrew; and Maes, Peter. 'Elevation and Cholera: an epidemiological spatial analysis of the cholera epidemic in Harare, Zimbabwe, 2008–2009'. Vol. 12, no. 442, 2012. https://doi.org/10.1186/1471-2458-12-442.

Mahase, Elisabeth. 'Covid-19: was the decision to delay the UK's lockdown over fears of "behavioural fatigue" based on evidence?' *BMJ*. 2020;370:m3166 https://www.bmj.com/content/370/bmj.m3166.

Mallapaty, Smriti. 'Antibody Tests Suggest that Coronavirus Infections Vastly Exceed Official Counts'. *Nature.* 2020-04-17.

Mancini, Donato Paolo. 'UK Spending on Covid Vaccines Hits Nearly £12bn, Watchdog Says'. *Financial Times.* 2020-12-16.

Mattsson, Anna. 'Tror du att du smittats av viruset — gör så här' (If you think you've been infected by the virus — here's what to do). *TT News Agency.* 2020-03-01.

McKenzie, F. Ellis. 'Smallpox Models as Policy Tools.' *Emerging Infectious Diseases.* Vol. 10, no. 11, 2004: 2044–2047. doi:10.3201/eid1011.040455

Medin, Joakim. 'Från förebild till värsting — Ungerns tio år under Orbán' (From role model to ruffian). *Utrikesmagasinet.* 2020-05-28.

Mellgren, Fredrik. 'Belgisk professor i SVT: Flockimmunitet dröjer' (Belgian professor in Sweden's Television: herd immunity will be a long time coming). *Svenska Dagbladet.* 2020-05-17.

Morabia Alfredo. 'Epidemiology's 350th Anniversary: 1662-2012'. *Epidemiology.* Vol. 24, no. 2, 2013: 179–83.

Nilsson, Johan. 'Därför sprids coronaviruset i kluster' (Why the coronavirus spreads in clusters). *TT News Agency / Ny Teknik.* 2020-06-26.

———. 'Överdödligheten 2020 tyder på lägre dödstal i covid-19' (2020 excess mortality indicates lower Covid-19 death toll). *TT News Agency.* 2021-01-13.

Nilsson, P.M. 'Klimatet har fått nytt pris' (New price tag on climate). *Dagens Industri.* 2019-10-11.

Nordenskiöld, Tomas and Strömberg, Maggie. 'Doldisen leder Löfvens krisgrupp — "som ett krig"' (Hidden figure leads Löfven's crisis group — "like a war"). *Expressen.* 2020-04-05.

Obminska, Ania. 'Det mest överraskande var hur oförberedda vi var' (Biggest surprise: how unprepared we were). *Ny Teknik.* 2020-06-05.

Olsen, Björn. *Pandemi: myterna, fakta, hoten* (Pandemic: myths, facts, threats). Norstedts, 2010.

Olterman, Philip. 'Angela Merkel Draws on Science Background in Covid-19 Explainer'. *The Guardian.* 2020-04-16.

Ottosson, Alexander; Palm, Emilia; and Wide, Erica. 'Centrum för rättvisa: "Coronapandemin och grundlagen — är grundlagen hinder för hårdare restriktioner?"' (Centre for Justice: 'The Covid pandemic and the constitution — is the constitution an obstacle for tougher restrictions?'). 2020-12-10.

Payne, Adam and Colson, Thomas. 'Boris Johnson Took Advice from Sweden's

No-Lockdown Scientist Before Rejecting Tougher Coronavirus Restrictions'. *Business Insider*. 2020-09-24.

Persson, Ulf and Olofsson, Sara. 'Ett QALY är värt mer än två miljoner kronor' (One QALY worth more than 2 million SEK). *Läkartidningen*. 2018-08-20.

Phillips, Nicky. 'The Coronavirus Is Here to Stay — Here's What That Means'. *Nature*. 2020-02-16.

Pnajwani, Abbas. 'Why This Poll Gives a Misleading View on How Many People the Public Think Covid-19 Has Killed'. *Full Fact*. 2020-08-05.

Quammen, David. *Spillover: animal infections and the next human pandemic*. W. W. Norton and Company, 2013.

Reimegård, Lisa. 'Inte motiverat att vaccinera pojkar mot HPV' (Vaccinating boys against HPV not justified). *LäkemedelsVärlden*. 2009-10-12.

Richtel, Matt. *An Elegant Defense*. Newbury House Publishers, 2019.

Rogvall, Filippa. 'Olsen: Fullt möjligt att stoppa coronaviruset' (Olsen: completely possible to stop the coronavirus). *Expressen*. 2021-02-23.

Rohrbasser, Jean-Marc. 'Les Hasards de la Variole' (The hazards of smallpox). *Astérion. Philosophie, histoire des idées, pensée politique*, Vol. 9, 2011.

Rydén, Daniel. 'Krav på munskydd på kollektivtrafiken i Danmark' (Mask mandate on public transport in Denmark). *Sydsvenskan*. 2020-08-18.

Sencer, D.J.; Dull, H.B.; and Langmuir, A.D. 'Epidemiologic Basis for Eradication of Measles in 1967'. *Public Health Reports*. Vol. 82, no. 3, 1967: 253–56.

Skogelin, Marc. 'Tretton personer smittade i Sverige' (Thirteen people infected in Sweden). *Aftonbladet*. 2020-02-29.

Sokonicki, Amanda. 'Regeringen kan inte fortsätta ducka — coronakrisen är på allvar' (Government can't keep ducking — the Covid crisis is serious). *Dagens Nyheter*. 2020-03-01.

Solås Suvatne, Steinar. 'Sa ifra i lukket Erna-møte' (Put her foot down in closed Erna meeting). *Dagbladet*. 2020-04-23.

Steerpike. 'Six Questions That Neil Ferguson Should Be Asked'. *The Spectator*. 2020-04-16.

Stenberg, Eva. 'Myndigheternas information om coronaviruset är förvirrande' (Confusing information from authorities about coronavirus). *Dagens Nyheter*. 2020-03-03.

Strittmatter, Kai. 'Das nächste Ischgl' (The next Ischgl). *Süddeutsche Zeitung*. 2020-03-22.

Strömberg, Maggie and Nilsson, Torbjörn. 'Så blev coronatesterna vårens stora stridsfråga' (How Covid tests became the contentious issue of the spring). *Expressen*. 2020-05-16.

Sturcke, James. 'Bird Flu Pandemic Could Kill 150m'. *The Guardian*. 2005-09-30.

Svahn, Claes and Hallgren, Magnus. 'Tegnells förklaring: Därför dog så många tidigt i Sverige' (Tegnell's explanation: why so many died early in Sweden). *Dagens Nyheter*. 2020-09-17.

Syal, Rajeev. 'No Evidence £22bn Test-and-Trace Scheme Cut Covid Rates in England, Say MPs'. *The Guardian*. 2021-03-10.

Søndergaard, Morten. 'Professor i Sydkorea: Då misslyckas Sveriges taktik' (Professor in South Korea: when Sweden's tactics fail). *Svenska Dagbladet*. 2020-04-26.

Tegnell, Anders. 'The Epidemiology and Consequences of Wound Infections Caused by Coagulase Negative Staphylococci After Thoracic Surgery'. Dissertation. Linköping University, 2002.

Topley, W.W.C. and Wilson, G.S. 'The Spread of Bacterial Infection. The Problem of Herd-Immunity'. *The Journal of Hygiene*. Vol. 21, no. 3, 1923: 243–49. doi:10.1017/s0022172400031478.

Torén, Kjell. 'Svag evidens för att munskydd minskar smitta hos allmänhet' (Weak evidence to indicate face masks reduce transmission among the public). *Läkartidningen*. 2020-08-24.

Turborn, Erik. 'Umeåforskare kritiseras för debattartikel — "Det har blivit en pseudodebatt" (Umeå scientists criticised for op-ed — 'it's turned into a pseudo debate'). *Västerbottens-Kuriren*. 2020-04-17.

Tångeberg, Johannes; Uggla, Simon; Sundberg, Roger; and Persson, Jimmy. 'Äldre nekas sjukhusvård under pandemin' (Elderly denied hospital care during the pandemic). *Eskilstuna-Kuriren*. 2020-05-12.

von Schreeb, Johan. 'Wolodarski undergräver svensk expertis' (Wolodarski undermines Swedish expertise). *Svenska Dagbladet*. 2020-03-16.

Wang, Cindy; Ellis, Samsom; and Bloomberg. 'How Taiwan's Covid Response Became the World's Envy'. *Fortune*. 2020-10-31.

Westin, Adam. 'Därför ville Tegnell inte prata om "andra vågen"' (Here's why Tegnell didn't want to talk about 'second wave'). *Aftonbladet*. 2020-11-24.

Westman Svenselius, Monica. 'OECD-ländernas politiker tar efter varandra' (OECD countries' politicians take after each other). Linköping University. 2020-08-12.

Whipple, Tom. 'Coronavirus Vaccine Trial May Need to Infect People'. *The Times*. 2020-05-29.

Whitehead, Margaret. 'William Farr's Legacy to the Study of Inequalities in Health'. *Bulletin of the World Health Organization*, 2000.

Winter, Carin, ed. 'Statens Bakteriologiska Laboratorium 1909–1993' (The National Bacteriological Laboratory, 1909–1993). Stockholm: Statens bakteriologiska laboratorium, 1993.

Woodward, Bob. *Rage*. Simon & Schuster, 2020.

Wright, Lawrence. 'The Plague Year: the mistakes and the struggles behind America's coronavirus tragedy'. *The New Yorker*. 2020-12-28.

Wu, Joseph T.; Leung, Kathy; and Leung, Gabriel M. 'Nowcasting and Forecasting the Potential Domestic and International Spread of the 2019-nCoV Outbreak Originating in Wuhan, China: a modelling study'. *The Lancet*. Vol. 395, no. 10225, 2020: 689–97.

Zhong, Raymond and Mozur, Paul. 'To Tame Coronavirus, Mao-Style Social Control Blankets China'. *The New York Times*. 2020-02-15.

Åbom, Per-Erik. *Farsoter och epidemier: En historisk odyssé från pest till ebola* (Contagions and epidemics: a historical odyssey from the plague to ebola). Atlantis, 2015.

Örtengren, Emanuel. 'Stabsläge är det nya normala i vården' (State of heightened preparedness the new normal within healthcare services). Tankesmedjan Timbro. 2020-02-25.

'Fewer Than 20,000 In Anti-Dry Parade: slogans from Bible.' *New York Times*. 5 July 1921, author not named.

Radio / TV

BBC News. 'WHO Head: "Our Key Message Is: Test, Test, Test."' 2020-03-16.

Channel 4 News. 'UK Moves to "Delay" Phase for "Worst Public Health Crisis for a Generation"'. YouTube. 2020-03-20.

Djurberg, Björn. 'Xi Jinping besökte Wuhan för första gången' (Xi Jinping visits Wuhan for the first time). Sveriges Radio. 2020-03-10.

France 24. 'France Extends Weekend Lockdown to Northern Pas-de-Calais Region'. 2021-03-06.

Hedtjärn, Erik; Rosén, Emelie; and Öhman, Daniel. 'När 22 forskare underkände Sveriges coronastrategi' (When 22 scientists gave Sweden's Covid strategy a failing grade). *Ekot granskar.* Sveriges Radio. 2020-04-26.

RTE. 'Finland to Begin Three-Week Lockdown on 8 March'. 2021-02-25.

SVT Nyheter. 'Anders Tegnell: Vi har haft en mer omfattande första våg' (Anders Tegnell: we've had a more extensive first wave). 2020-05-10.

SVT Nyheter. 'Coronakommissionen: Misslyckats att skydda Sveriges äldre' (Covid-19 commission: failure to protect Sweden's elderly). 2020-12-15.

SVT Nyheter. 'Experter kritiserar Anders Tegnell i mejldiskussion' (Experts criticise Anders Tegnell in email thread). 2020-03-19.

SVT Nyheter. 'Forskargrupp: Så många kan hamna i intensivvård' (Scientist Group: this many could end up in intensive care). 2020-03-20.

SVT Nyheter. 'Statsepidemiologen: "Stabil situation i Sverige"' (State Epidemiologist: 'stable situation in Sweden'). 2020-03-25.

SVT Nyheter. 'Se hur matematikprofessorn räknar ut när Stockholm uppnår flockimmunitet' (Watch a mathematics professor calculate when Stockholm reaches herd immunity). 2020-04-20.

SVT Nyheter. 'Hösten blev värre än Folkhälsomyndighetens värsta scenario' (The autumn turned out worse than Public Health Agency's worst-case scenario). 2020-12-18.

Sveriges Radio. 'Söndagsintervjun: Johan Giesecke — om pappa, pandemier och popularitet' (The Sunday Interview: Johan Giesecke — about dad, pandemics, and popularity). 2020-08-30.

Sveriges Radio. 'Behöver grundlagen skrivas om för att hantera en pandemi?' (Does the constitution need to be rewritten to handle a pandemic?). 2020-11-21.

Tegnell, Anders. 'Sommar i P1' (Summer in P1). Sveriges Radio. 2020-06-24.

TV4-nyheterna. 'Därför väljer Anders Tegnell cykeln till tv4-huset' (Here's why Anders Tegnell takes the bike to the TV4 building). 2020-12-11.

Internet

Bank, Justin. 'Palin vs. Obama: death panels'. *FactCheck.org*. 2009-08-14. http://www.factcheck.org/2009/08/palin-vs-obama-death-panels,

Cabinet Office. 'Coronavirus: How to Stay Safe and Help Prevent the Spread'. GOV.UK. 2021-03-29. https://www.gov.uk/guidance/national-lockdown-stay-at-home.

Comparisons of all-cause mortality between European countries and regions: data up to week ending 3 September 2021. ons.gov.uk/peoplepopulationandcommunity/birthsdeathsandmarriages/deaths/datasets/comparisonsofallcausemortalitybetweeneuropeancountries andregions, reuters.com/article/us-health-coronavirus-europe-mortality-idUSKBN2BG1R9

ECDC. 'Using Face Masks in the Community: first update — effectiveness in reducing transmission of Covid-19'. 2021-02-15. https://www.ecdc.europa.eu/en/publications-data/using-face-masks-community-reducing-covid-19-transmission.

Engström, Mats. 'Regeringen släppte rodret när EU diskuterade munskydd' (Government let go of the rudder when EU discussed face masks). 2020-11-22. http://mengstrom.blogspot.com/2020/11/regeringen-slappte-rodret-nar-eu.html.

Euractiv. '"We Are at War": France postpones second round of elections, pension reform'. 2020-03-17. https://www.euractiv.com/section/elections/news/we-are-at-war-france-postpones-second-round-of-elections-pension-reform.

Folketinget. 'Rapport om myndighedernes håndtering af covid-19-pandemiens første fase' (Report on the authorities' handling of the first phase of the Covid-19 pandemic). 2021-01-29. https://www.ft.dk/da/aktuelt/nyheder/2021/01/udredning-om-covid_19.

Guardian News. 'Angela Merkel Uses Science Background in Coronavirus Explainer'. YouTube. 2020-04-16. https://www.youtube.com/watch?v=22SQVZ4CeXA&feature=emb_logo&ab_channel=GuardianNews.

Karlsten, Emanuel. 'Regeringen ändrade i dokument om coronastrategi — mening om kontrollerad spridning försvann' (Government changed document about Covid-19 strategy — sentence about controlled transmission disappeared). 2021-02-01. https://emanuelkarlsten.se/ regeringen-andrar-i-dokument-om-coronastrategi-raderar-mening-om-kontrollerad-spridning.

Ministry of Health and Social Affairs. 'Regleringsbrev för budgetåret 2020 avseende Folkhälsomyndigheten' (Appropriation directions for the fiscal year 2020 with respect to the Public Health Agency). The Swedish National Financial Management Authority. 2019-12-19. https://www.esv.se/statsliggaren/regleringsbrev/?rbid=20423,

———. 'Besöksförbudet på äldreboenden upphör 1 oktober' (Ban on nursing home visits ceases on 1 October). Government Offices of Sweden. 2020-09-15. https://www.regeringen.se/artiklar/2020/09/besoksforbudet-pa-aldreboenden-upphor-1-oktober.

———. 'Bemyndigande att underteckna en överenskommelse mellan staten och Sveriges Kommuner och Regioner om ökad nationell testning för covid-19' (Authorisation to sign an agreement between the State and Sweden's municipalities and regions about increased national testing for Covid-19). Government Offices of Sweden. 2020-11-19. https://www.regeringen.se/4ad3c7/contentassets/073ee870d0574feab0ffcad5b3d8d211/bemyndigande-att-underteckna-en-overenskommelse-mellan-staten-och-skr-om-okad-nationell-testning-for-covid-19_webb.pdf.

Ministry of Justice, Ministry of Culture. 'Förändringar i förordningen om förbud mot att hålla allmänna sammankomster och offentliga tillställningar' (Changes to the regulation on the prohibition on holding public gatherings and events). Government Offices of Sweden. 2020-10-22. https://www.regeringen.se/pressmeddelanden/2020/10/forandringar-i-forordningen-om-forbud-mot-att-halla-allmanna-sammankomster-och-offentliga-tillstallningar.

OECD. 'News Release: G20 GDP Growth Quarterly National Accounts — unprecedented falls in GDP in most G20 economies in second quarter of 2020'. 2020-09-14. https://www.oecd.org/sdd/na/g20-gdp-growth-second-quarter-2020-oecd.htm.

Office of Governor Gavin Newson. 'Governor Newsom Announces California Has Conducted Over 1 Million Diagnostic Tests for Covid-19 as Testing Capacity Ramps Up'. 2020-05-12. https://www.gov.ca.gov/2020/05/12/governor-newsom-announces-california-has-conducted-over-1-million-diagnostic-tests-for-covid-19-as-testing-capacity-ramps-up.

Public Health Agency of Sweden. 'Antal fall av covid-19 i Sverige' (Number of Covid-19 cases in Sweden). Updated daily. https://experience.arcgis.com/experience/09f821667ce64bf7be6f-9f87457ed9aa.

———. 'Uppdaterad riskbedömning för covid-19 i Sverige' (Updated risk assessment for Covid-19 in Sweden). 2020-03-02. https://www.folkhalsomyndigheten.se/nyheter-och-press/nyhetsarkiv/2020/mars/uppdaterad-riskbedomning-for-covid-19-i-sverige.

———. 'Pandemiberedskap. Hur vi förbereder oss — ett kunskapsunderlag' (Pandemic preparedness: how we prepare). 2012-12-19. https://www.folkhalsomyndigheten.se/publicerat-material/publikationsarkiv/p/pandemiberedskap-hur-vi-forbereder-oss-ett-kunskapsunderlag.

———. 'Skattning av peakdag och antal infekterade i covid-19-utbrottet i Stockholms län februari-april 2020' (Estimated peak day and number of infections during the Covid-19 outbreak in Stockholm County in February–April 2020). 2020-04-21. https://www.folkhalsomyndigheten.se/publicerat-material/publikationsarkiv/s/skattning-av-peakdag-och-antal-infekterade-i-covid-19-utbrottet-i-stockholms-lan-februari-april-2020.

———. 'Skattning av peakdag och antal infekterade i covid-19-utbrottet i Stockholms län februari-april 2020' (Estimated peak day and number of infections during the Covid-19 outbreak in Stockholm County in February–April 2020). 2020. https://www.folkhalsomyndigheten.se/contentassets/2da059f90b90458d8454a04955d1697f/skattning-peakdag-antal-infekterade-covid-19-utbrottet-stockholms-lan-februari-april-2020.pdf.

Riksdag (Sweden). 'Rekommendation om munskydd i kammare och kammarfoajé' (Recommendation on face masks in the chamber and chamber foyer). 2021-02-25. https://www.riksdagen.se/sv/aktuellt/2021/feb/25/rekommendation-om-munskydd-i-kammare-och-kammarfoaje.

———. 'Skriftlig fråga 2020/21:1630: Regeringens agerande avseende covid-19-pandemin' (Written query 2020/21:1630: the government's actions concerning the Covid-19 pandemic). 2021-02-04. https://www.riksdagen.se/sv/dokument-lagar/dokument/skriftlig-fraga/regeringens-agerande-avseende-covid-19-pandemin_H8111630.

Sokolnicki, Amanda [@A_Sokolnicki]. 'Tycker det är obegripligt att eleverna som nu kommer hem från sportlovsresor uppmanas gå till skolan på måndag — oavsett vilket land de varit i. Är som att Löfven i det här känsliga läget har outsourcat ansvaret att leda landet till Folkhälsomyndigheten' (Finding it incomprehensible that students now returning from trips over the February break are encouraged to go to school on Monday — regardless of what country they've been to. It's like Löfven in this sensitive situation has outsourced the responsibility to lead the country to the Public Health Agency.') Twitter. https://twitter.com/a_sokolnicki/status/1234036602499981312.

Statistics Sweden. 'GDP Indicator: sharp contraction in second quarter 2020'. 2020-08-05. https://www.scb.se/en/finding-statistics/statistics-by-subject-area/national-accounts/national-accounts/national-accounts-quarterly-and-annual-estimates/pong/statistical-news/national-accounts-second-quarter-2020

———. 'Döda i Sverige' (Swedish deaths). 2021-03-24. https://www.scb.se/hitta-statistik/sverige-i-siffror/manniskorna-i-sverige/doda-i-sverige.

Swedish Covid-19 Commission. 'Strategin att skydda de äldre har misslyckats' (The strategy to protect the elderly has failed). Swedish Government Official Reports. 2020-12-15. https://news.cision.com/se/coronakommissionen-s-2020-09/r/strategin-att-skydda-de-aldre-har-misslyckats,c3253192.

Times Higher Education. 'World University Rankings 2018'. https://www.timeshighereducation.com/world-university-rankings/2018/world-ranking#!/page/1/length/25/sort_by/rank/sort_order/asc/cols/stats.

Tyson, Alec and Maniam, Shiva. 'Behind Trump's Victory: divisions by race, gender, education'. Pew Research Center, 9 November 2016. https://www.pewresearch.org/fact-tank/2016/11/09/behind-trumps-victory-divisions-by-race-gender-education.

UNICEF. 'Across Virtually Every Key Measure of Childhood, Progress Has Gone Backward, UNICEF Says as Pandemic Declaration Hits One-Year Mark'. 2021-03-10. https://www.unicef.org/press-releases/across-virtually-every-key-measure-childhood-progress-has-gone-backward-unicef-says.

Walker, Shaun and Smith, Helena. 'Why has eastern Europe suffered less from coronavirus than the west?' theguardian.com/world/2020/may/05

World Bank. 'Covid-19 to Add as Many as 150 Million Extreme Poor by 2021'. 2020-10-07. https://www.worldbank.org/en/news/press-release/2020/10/07/covid-19-to-add-as-many-as-150-million-extreme-poor-by-2021.

World Health Organization. 'Global>China.' https://covid19.who.int/region/wpro/country/cn.

———. 'Pandemic Influenza Risk Management'. 2017. https://www.who.int/influenza/preparedness/pandemic/PIRM_update_052017.pdf.